DIRTY, LAZY, KETO

FAST FOOD GUIDE:

10 Carbs or Less

William & Stephanie

Laska

DIRTY, LAZY, KETO

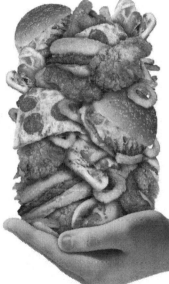

FAST FOOD GUIDE »

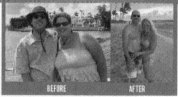

BEFORE   AFTER

10 CARBS OR LESS

WILLIAM LASKA & STEPHANIE LASKA, M.ED

For additional resources, visit the author website:

http://DirtyLazyKeto.com

You may contact or follow the author on social media:

https://twitter.com/140lost
https://instagram.com/140lost/
https://facebook.com/dirtylazyketo

Join other fans of the DIRTY, LAZY, KETO community by joining the FREE author-led Facebook group:

https://facebook.com/groups/DirtyLazyKeto

First Edition

Cover designed by Alerrandre

DEDICATION

I would like to dedicate <u>DIRTY, LAZY, KETO Fast Food Guide: 10 Carbs or Less</u> to our road warrior children. On our hundreds of weekend adventures, they have learned to fuel themselves off of the value menus at fast food restaurants across this great nation. Our family operates on a tight budget, but we still believe in getting out of the house to see the world!

Just because we started eating healthier to lose weight doesn't mean we stopped enjoying fast food restaurants. Over a two-year period, Stephanie lost 140 pounds while Bill trimmed off 40 pounds. Despite being frequent eaters of fast food (a few times a week), both Stephanie and Bill reduced their cholesterol by over a hundred points - EACH!

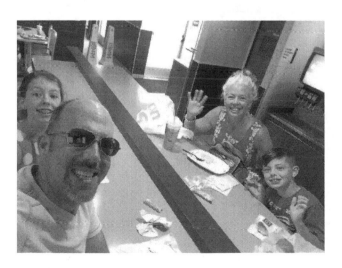

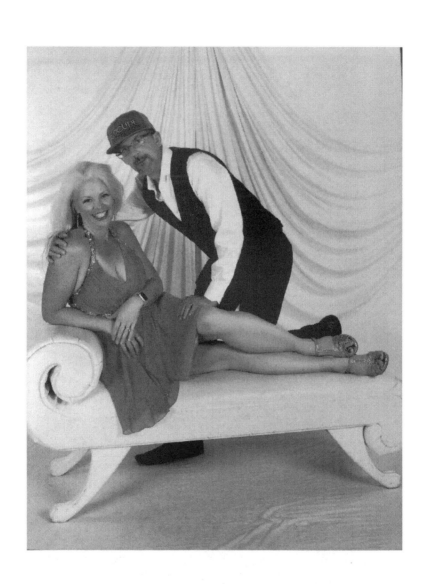

ACKNOWLEDGEMENTS

When our new books come out, we often give them away for FREE or at a super reduced price to our loyal fans, so don't miss out! REGISTER: www.http://eepurl.com/dFE7wv

DIRTY, LAZY, KETO Fast Food Guide: 10 Carbs or Less is the second in a series of publications meant to help support your path to better health. More topics to come!

We are constantly updating our website with tips, articles, and support for the keto dieter. Be sure to check us out for the latest info at www.http://dirtylazyketo.com

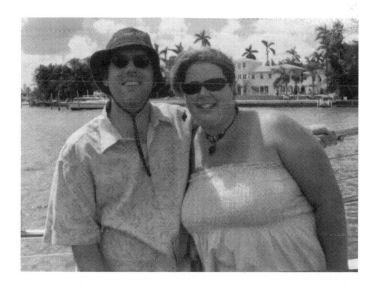

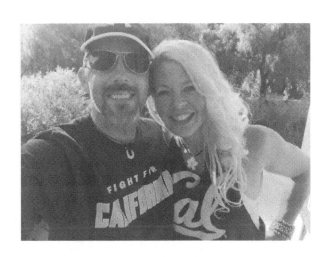

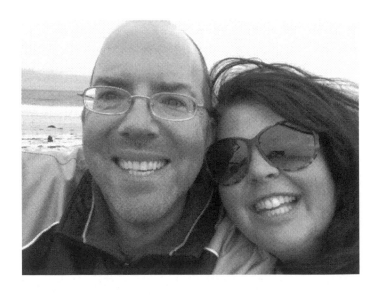

CHARITY

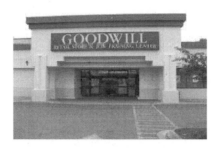

Proceeds from the DIRTY, LAZY, KETO book series benefit one of my favorite charities, Goodwill Industries International, Inc. The Goodwlll helps people with barriers to employment by giving them a second chance. I feel like I have been given a second chance at life after losing 140 pounds, so this mission statement resonates with me!

Over a year and a half, I dropped about ten pounds a month. My clothes, at times, were literally falling off of me. I know that sounds like a good problem to have, right? Who doesn't love shopping? (#firstworldproblems) The reality is that buying an entirely new wardrobe every month came with a hefty price tag. My wallet literally could not support my weight loss! Buying clothes at the Goodwill helped me transition through eleven sizes in clothes. I went from a size 26 down to a 4/6. That's a lot of clothes, people!

Thank you for helping me support Goodwill by spreading the word about <u>DIRTY, LAZY, KETO Fast Food Guide: 10 Carbs or Less</u>. Something simple YOU can do to help is to leave an honest Amazon review. Reviews on Amazon help the book get noticed by other readers. Thank you for your help!

Table of Contents

BACKGROUND: WHAT IS DIRTY, LAZY, KETO? 1

IN DEFENSE OF FAST FOOD 6

BENEFITS OF DIRTY, LAZY, KETO FAST FOOD GUIDE: 10 CARBS OR LESS 12

1. COFFEE 15

COFFEE HACKS FROM DIRTY, LAZY, KETO: 16

STARBUCKS: HACKS FROM THE AUTHORS OF DIRTY, LAZY, KETO 18

STARBUCKS: 10 CARBS OR LESS 21

DUNKIN' DONUTS: HACKS FROM THE AUTHORS OF DIRTY, LAZY, KETO 37

DUNKIN' DONUTS: 10 CARBS OR LESS 39

MCDONALD'S MCCAFÉ: HACKS FROM THE AUTHORS OF DIRTY, LAZY, KETO 48

MCDONALD'S MCCAFÉ: 10 CARBS OR LESS 51

2. BURGERS 55

BURGER HACKS FROM DIRTY, LAZY, KETO: 56

MCDONALD'S: HACKS FROM THE AUTHORS OF DIRTY, LAZY, KETO 58

MCDONALD'S: 10 CARBS OR LESS 60

BURGER KING: HACKS FROM THE AUTHORS OF DIRTY, LAZY, KETO 62

BURGER KING: 10 CARBS OR LESS 64

WENDY'S: HACKS FROM THE AUTHORS OF DIRTY, LAZY, KETO 66

WENDY'S: 10 CARBS OR LESS 67

DAIRY QUEEN: HACKS FROM THE AUTHORS OF DIRTY, LAZY, KETO 69

DAIRY QUEEN: 10 CARBS OR LESS 70

IN-N-OUT: HACKS FROM THE AUTHORS OF DIRTY, LAZY, KETO 72

IN-N-OUT: 10 CARBS OR LESS 73

JACK IN THE BOX: HACKS FROM THE AUTHORS OF DIRTY, LAZY, KETO 75

JACK IN THE BOX: 10 CARBS OR LESS 76

CARL'S JR./HARDEE'S: HACKS FROM THE AUTHORS OF DIRTY, LAZY, KETO 78

CARL'S JR./HARDEE'S: 10 CARBS OR LESS 80

FIVE GUYS: HACKS FROM THE AUTHORS OF DIRTY, LAZY, KETO 83

FIVE GUYS: 10 CARBS OR LESS 85

WHATABURGER: HACKS FROM THE AUTHORS OF DIRTY, LAZY, KETO 87

WHATABURGER: 10 CARBS OR LESS   88

3.   MEXICAN   91

MEXICAN FOOD HACKS FROM THE AUTHORS OF DIRTY, LAZY, KETO
    92
TACO BELL: HACKS FROM THE AUTHORS OF DIRTY, LAZY, KETO   93
TACO BELL: 10 CARBS OR LESS   95
DEL TACO: HACKS FROM THE AUTHORS OF DIRTY, LAZY, KETO   98
DEL TACO: 10 CARBS OR LESS   99
CHIPOTLE: HACKS FROM THE AUTHORS OF DIRTY, LAZY, KETO   101
CHIPOTLE: 10 CARBS OR LESS   103
EL POLLO LOCO: HACKS FROM THE AUTHORS OF DIRTY, LAZY, KETO
    105
EL POLLO LOCO: 10 CARBS OR LESS   106

4.SANDWICHES   109

SANDWICH HACKS FROM DIRTY, LAZY, KETO: 110
SUBWAY: HACKS FROM THE AUTHORS OF DIRTY, LAZY, KETO   111
SUBWAY: 10 CARBS OR LESS   113
QUIZNO'S: HACKS FROM THE AUTHORS OF DIRTY, LAZY, KETO   117
QUIZNO'S: 10 CARBS OR LESS   118
PANERA BREAD: HACKS FROM THE AUTHORS OF DIRTY, LAZY, KETO
    120
PANERA BREAD: 10 CARBS OR LESS   122
JIMMY JOHN'S: HACKS FROM THE AUTHORS OF DIRTY, LAZY, KETO 125
JIMMY JOHN'S: 10 CARBS OR LESS   126
JERSEY MIKE'S: HACKS FROM THE AUTHORS OF DIRTY, LAZY, KETO 128
JERSEY MIKE'S: 10 CARBS OR LESS   129
SONIC DRIVE IN: HACKS FROM THE AUTHORS OF DIRTY, LAZY, KETO
    131
SONIC DRIVE IN: 10 CARBS OR LESS   132
ARBY'S: HACKS FROM THE AUTHORS OF DIRTY, LAZY, KETO   135
ARBY'S: 10 CARBS OR LESS   137
JAMBA JUICE: HACKS FROM THE AUTHORS OF DIRTY, LAZY, KETO   139
JAMBA JUICE: 10 CARBS OR LESS   141

4.   CHICKEN   143

CHICKEN HACKS FROM DIRTY, LAZY, KETO: 144
CHICK-FIL-A: HACKS FROM THE AUTHORS OF DIRTY, LAZY, KETO   145
CHICK-FIL-A: 10 CARBS OR LESS   147
KFC: HACKS FROM THE AUTHORS OF DIRTY, LAZY, KETO   150

KFC: 10 Carbs or Less   151
Popeyes: Hacks from the Authors of DIRTY, LAZY, KETO   153
Popeyes: 10 Carbs or Less   154
Church's: Hacks from the Authors of DIRTY, LAZY, KETO   156
Church's: 10 Carbs or Less   158
Wing Stop: Hacks from the Authors of DIRTY, LAZY, KETO   160
Wing Stop: 10 Carbs or Less   161
Buffalo Wild Wings: Hacks from the Authors of DIRTY, LAZY,
KETO   163
Buffalo Wild Wings: 10 Carbs or Less   164

5.   CHINESE   167

Chinese Food Hacks From DIRTY, LAZY, KETO: 168
Panda Express: Hacks from the Authors of DIRTY, LAZY, KETO
                                                                 169
Panda Express: 10 Carbs or Less   170
Ono Hawaiian BBQ: Hacks from the Authors of DIRTY, LAZY,
KETO   172
Ono Hawaiian BBQ: 10 Carbs or Less   174

6.   PIZZA   177

Pizza Hacks From DIRTY, LAZY, KETO: 178
Fat Head Pizza Crust   180
Little Caesars: Hacks from the Authors of DIRTY, LAZY, KETO
                                                                 182
Little Caesars: 10 Carbs or Less   183
Domino's Pizza: Hacks from the Authors of DIRTY, LAZY, KETO
                                                                 185
Domino's: 10 Carbs or Less   187
Pizza Hut: Hacks from the Authors of DIRTY, LAZY, KETO   189
Pizza Hut: 10 Carbs or Less   191

7.   SEAFOOD   193

Seafood Hacks From DIRTY, LAZY, KETO   194
Long John Silver's: Hacks from the Authors of DIRTY, LAZY,
KETO   195
Long John Silver's: 10 Carbs or Less   196

8.   FINAL WORDS   199

Background: What is Dirty, Lazy, Keto?

What is DIRTY, LAZY, KETO and how is this different from a traditional ketogenic diet?

> *Sometimes a girl just needs a Diet Coke®.*
> *Please don't call the keto police!*

DIRTY, LAZY, KETO was only inspired by the ketogenic diet. It is not a strict interpretation. It offers the reader a unique approach to weight loss that Stephanie found helped her to lose 140 pounds and maintain the weight loss for going on five years. Bam!

> *I don't know about you, but I'm tired of the weight loss merry-go-round. I want to figure this out NOW and make this a LONG-TERM solution.*

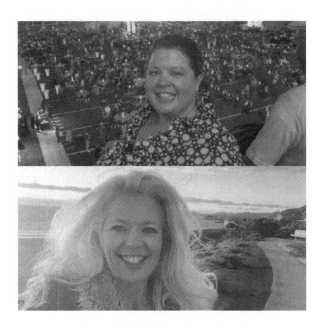

Unlike DIRTY, LAZY, KETO, the traditional ketogenic diet tends to be very strict. Usually, strict keto adheres to a twenty carbs per day rule. Artificial sweeteners like Splenda® are frowned upon by the strict keto police, so fat bombs, Diet Coke®, and HALO® ice cream are definitely out of the question (who invited THAT guy to the party?). Of course, I'm speaking generally here. I'm sure there are exceptions, but that's pretty much the gist of strict keto. Traditionalists often take their keto commitment to the next level by monitoring not only their intake of fat, carbohydrate, and protein grams, but also count calories. Many find success with this method but NOT the authors, Stephanie and William Laska. They feel differently, and want to offer an alternative for those that might agree.

Is a strict keto lifestyle realistic or sustainable long-term? Many feel they need to tweak the rules in order to find dieting success. Personally, I could never follow such rigid guidelines! Not everyone has the budget or lifestyle that supports organic vegetable shopping. Eating grass-fed beef and Irish butter won't give you an advantage in the weight loss challenge.

> *Throwing money at your weight loss problem won't fix it any faster. If that was the case, then Oprah would be skinny. Let's get real here.*

Lazy keto followers believe in the science of keto, but say to hell with all that tracking business. Before you rush to any judgement, understand these folks can be just as successful as strict keto. Lazy keto doesn't mean they are relaxing by the pool somewhere. Rather, "lazy" is just a coined term that describes a way of focusing on carb count only (not fat, protein or calories). Lazy keto dieters usually aren't documenting every bite they eat with some little calculator or app. In general, lazy keto followers choose lower carb, higher fat foods to enjoy while staying "under" or "around" their carb goals/limits for the day.

So, what is all this "dirty" business about? Is there some X-rated version of keto out there in cyberspace? (Probably). Oh, we are a fun group, but not THAT kind of fun. Dirty keto dieters like to break the rules now and again with our ingredient choices. We are wild and crazy in that regard! We may not be strict, but... SURPRISE, we are sustainable and successful!

> *DIRTY, LAZY, KETO is open to using sugar and grain substitutes to make a recipe feel more "like we are used to" and not afraid of artificial anything, including FAST FOOD!*

So that's what DIRTY, LAZY, KETO is all about. We eat low carb. We lose weight. Got it?

There is no need to overcomplicate our eating, in my opinion. Counting fat, counting protein, counting calories… where does it end? That's enough counting to make me feel like a crazy person. I worry that overcommitting yourself to so much counting might lead

3

to rebellion or exhaustion. In the short term that strategy might be effective, but for the rest of your life? I don't think that is going to work forever. I imagine you want to lose weight and keep it off forever, so a long-term strategy is required.

Focusing on the daily carb count has "been enough" in my experience with weight loss. By limiting my daily intake to a range of 20-50 carbs (this varies according to your activity level and body mass), I've lost 140 pounds and maintained my weight loss for five years. I believe one can be successful at losing weight without tracking every macronutrient.

If you would like to explore this topic in detail, you might enjoy reading the first book of the DIRTY, LAZY, KETO series. That's where all the nitty-gritty is discussed.

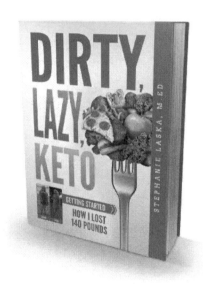

Learn how you can "have your keto cake and eat it too" in Stephanie's best-selling Amazon book, DIRTY, LAZY, KETO Getting Started: How I Lost 140 Pounds. Stephanie explains with great detail and humor WHY this way of eating works so well for her and even includes what foods she recommends. It's a must read!

Enough jibber jabber now. Let's get serious about fast food!

In Defense of Fast Food

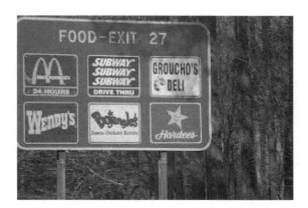

We have all been there. We are out on the road when suddenly, the HANGER creeps up and we need to eat, like RIGHT NOW. Perhaps in an alternative, perfect universe, we would've planned ahead and packed a bag of "all natural, earth-friendly, locally grown" keto snacks. For most of us, that's just not realistic. We lead busy lives, work long hours and are constantly on the move. Between commuting to work or getting kids to activities, we are all overscheduled and could use a break.

> *Many, if not all of us, grew up being told that fast food was unhealthy. Well, a lot has changed over the years! Many of these restaurants have drastically improved their menus.*

The reality is that for most of us, fast food is an integral part of our existence. Whether your motives stem from cost, convenience, or even just pleasure, I support your lifestyle to eat on the run. There is no judgment here. I do the same thing! I want to assure you that it is possible to eat fast food while enjoying the DIRTY, LAZY, KETO diet. It is 100% possible to eat fast food *while still losing weight*!

To be clear, I'm not getting all "Jared" on you (remember the Subway spokesman? We all know how THAT turned out!). This book is not recommending you go to fast food for every meal for the rest of your life. I'm pretty sure that common sense would suggest otherwise. But, for all the keto critics out there, I need to state the obvious: Eating at home is probably healthier!

> *This guide is meant to educate you about making informed decisions while eating fast food, because WE ALL EAT FAST FOOD!*

Now that we've acknowledged eating fast food can be part of our diet, let's drill down to specifics. I don't want you making excuses (ignorance is bliss) or blindly picking what "looks healthy" on the menu. That beautiful salad shown in neon lights on the drive thru sign might be littered with candied nuts, sugar filled dressing, and breaded protein. No more excuses, my friend. Let's get real about the choices we are making.

> *I'm going to ask you a personal question here... Have you ever "BURIED THE EVIDENCE?"*

Have you ever thrown your fast food trash away (before coming home) so your family wouldn't know you stopped for a bite to eat? Have you ever pulled into the garage and quickly "hid" your wrappers in the trash can (carefully piling fresh garbage on top of the wrappers to literally AND figuratively BURY THE EVIDENCE!)?

Well I am going to admit to doing both of these guilt-ridden behaviors. I'm sure I'm not alone here! Anyone else? Anyone? *(Oh, that's so embarrassing if I am the only one.)*

The shame of eating fast food needs to stop. I'm not a bad person because I like to grab something quick once in a while. The convenience of a drive thru will never, ever, lose its appeal. I don't care how fancy you are!

Furthermore, acknowledging that fast food is part of my diet is downright liberating. I'm not going to be one of "those people" that claim NEVER to eat fast food. "Girl, stop your lyin'," is what I want to say to THOSE people.

There is a shame/guilt/overeat cycle associated with fast food. Combined with eating in secret, this leads to PROBLEMS! I am going to be LOUD AND PROUD about eating fast food, but also promise to educate myself to order wisely. No more excuses!

Are you getting excited now? I bet you have a lot of questions bubbling up. Which fast food restaurants are best for keto in terms of cost and convenience? Who offers menu choices that are affordable and filling, but most important, low in carbs? Is it possible to order a sandwich and stay on plan? What are my options here? Let's dig down and answer these questions in an easy to read and simple format.

> *I want to EMPOWER YOU with information so YOU can make better choices for YOURSELF.*

While researching fast food restaurants for hundreds of hours, several things became clear to me. First, DAMN that made me hungry! Second, it become obvious right away that even though the government requires fast food restaurants to share their nutrition information, it's not always easy for a consumer to find that information. In fact, sometimes it's downright HIDDEN!

An example of "sneakiness" that comes to mind is about a certain restaurant chain that serves a lot of cheesecake (can you guess which one?). For YEARS, their website didn't offer nutrition information about the menu. Rather, they required a customer ask for that paperwork in person at the restaurant. REALLY? What were they trying to hide? Are they embarrassed about the carb count in their cheesecake? (Um, probably!) Furthermore, once I drove to the restaurant and asked for their nutrition guide I found that it was printed in like size 6 font. I had to use my iPhone camera as a magnifying glass just to read that sucker! Bottom line, this info is not easy to find. (Please don't ban me dear cheesecake restaurant, I love your low carb cheesecake!)[1]

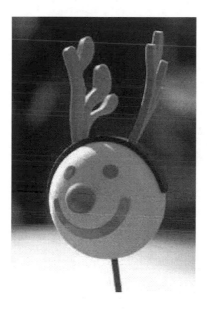

Gathering this data is not a novel idea. There are many websites that have attempted such a gargantuan task, but none as thorough, complete, and entertaining as <u>DIRTY, LAZY, KETO Fast Food Guide: 10 Carbs or Less</u>!

---

[1] I must not have been the only complainer. They recently published their nutrition info online. YEAH!

DIRTY, LAZY, KETO Fast Food Guide: 10 Carbs or Less is your one stop companion for weight loss on the go. No matter what fast food restaurant you find yourself at, this reference book will provide accurate nutrition information and suggestions to help you make informed choices.

> *By zeroing in on menu items that are less than 10 carbs, you can quickly decide what to order in the drive thru and avoid the guy behind you from honking his horn while you try to make up your mind.*

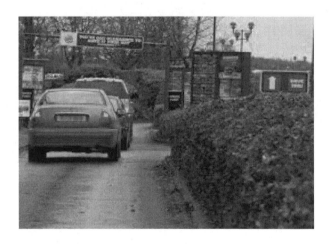

Disclaimer:

Sadly, not all fast food restaurants understand the keto or low carb diet. When restaurants provide nutrition information for a sandwich, for example, they often do not give the nutrition data if the bun is removed. The provided data is for the entire entrée, bun and all. In these situations, the authors used exhaustive research (literally hundreds of hours) to give their best estimation of carb count.

Additionally, because fast food entrees have different size buns (and tortillas) according to each unique sandwich, there is a slight variation to the carb count listed on their nutritional information website. For example ,the Filet-of-Fish® uses a different bun than a Big Mac®. The variety of buns have unique carb counts, and often are not clearly stated on the company website. Based on exhaustive research, the authors gave their best estimation of carb count.

As you conduct your own field research (enjoying fast food!) we hope you will help improve future editions by emailing us your discoveries and feedback at dirtylazyketo@gmail.com

All carbs listed throughout the guide are net carbs (total carbohydrates subtract fiber) when fiber grams are provided by the restaurant nutrition guide.

BENEFITS OF DIRTY, LAZY, KETO FAST FOOD GUIDE: 10 CARBS OR LESS

<u>DIRTY, LAZY, KETO Fast Food Guide: 10 Carbs or Less</u> EMPOWERS YOU to make healthier, guilt-free choices for YOURSELF.

- Prevents keto boredom! Discover NEW restaurants and NEW things to order
- Guilt-free ordering – You know EXACTLY what to order
- QUICK access – No irritating advertisements
- All in ONE spot – Easy to use and find what you're looking for
- 35 Fast Food and Coffee Restaurants explored!
- Hacks and Suggestions about WHAT and HOW to order
- Unique grading system – Author's Favorites? Earn GOLD STARS (or a SAD FACE!)
- HIDDEN and SECRET fast food menu options
- Hard to find links to interactive customizable nutrition guides
- Super entertaining commentary from your DIRTY, LAZY, KETO hosts
- Money-saving tips to stretch your low carb dollar
- BONUS: Fat Head Pizza Dough Recipe included!

"I live in the real world. I eat 'clean' foods when I can, but if I'm out running errands and get hungry, I'm going to grab a 'bunless' burger and not feel bad about it! I can find something to eat pretty much everywhere I go and still stay in ketosis. People can judge if they want, but the bottom line is that dirty or clean, keto works!"

– Carol M, Member of the DIRTY, LAZY, KETO Facebook Group

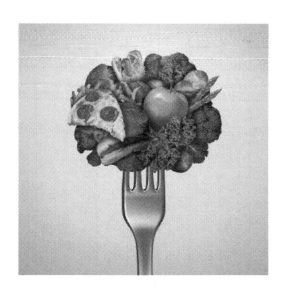

1. COFFEE

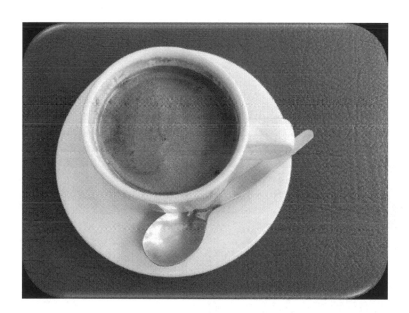

COFFEE HACKS From DIRTY, LAZY, KETO:

No matter what coffee chain you choose, try the following keto hacks:

*Ask the barista about the sugar-free sweeteners available, like the Torani brand of sugar-free syrups. If in doubt, order your coffee unsweetened AKA black, and be in control of your coffee with options that are available at the condiment bar.

*Don't be fooled by "sugar-free" or "skinny" in the menu titles as many of these options are still high in carbs! Be sure to check the website of your coffee house first for specifics (if not spelled out here).

*If you like a creamy coffee, order a splash of full cream (or half/half if cream isn't available). While this may be obvious to the experienced keto dieter, new folks might be surprised that cream has less carbs than low fat milk or nonfat milk. If you prefer a dairy alternative, unsweetened almond milk is a recommended choice and commonly available at coffee bars.

*Be sure to stress the word "splash" if asking for cream. Baristas are trained to provide a beverage that "tastes good" but not necessarily one that's healthy. Like any good businessperson, baristas also want your drink to also "look good" and may apply a certain amount of dairy to your drink to accomplish this. Be assertive about the quantity of cream you want in your drink.

*Consider asking for "1/2 full cream and 1/2 steamed water" to reduce the heavy-handed pour.

*Omit the whipped cream (the canned stuff) or enjoy a teeny, tiny bit to be wild and crazy.

*When ordering a snack, always go "breadless" or "wrap-less".

*There are literally THOUSANDS of unique combinations you could order at a coffee house, so we highlight the most popular coffee drinks to help you get started. We apologize if your exact drink is not listed and have provided the nutrition link directly to the restaurant for situations like this.

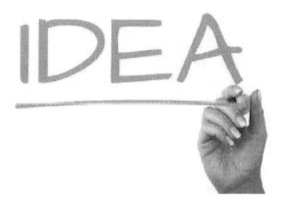

STARBUCKS: HACKS FROM THE AUTHORS OF DIRTY, LAZY, KETO

Stephanie recommends keeping a close eye on how much whipping cream is in your coffee. A little bit goes a long way! In her opinion,

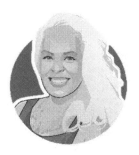

the number one reason people stall on the keto diet usually comes down to Starbucks, and the sweeteners and cream are the lurking evil culprit. Because baristas are often heavy-handed with the cream, ask for it *in a separate cup*. That way you can control the amount in your coffee. **NO excuses!**

Many of us have a regular habit of visiting Starbucks. It's hard to break the habit of stopping at Starbucks on the way to work. Instead of buying yourself a fancy drink, have you considered buying a "coffee tote" to bring to work/social events? The cost is around $12, and you walk away with a full coffee bar for everyone to enjoy.

Because most of your drinks here are caffeinated, Stephanie recommends ordering an extra-large ice water (complimentary) with every coffee drink you order. Caffeinated drinks are dehydrating!

Bill has a lot to say about Starbucks. There are drinks here that have over a hundred carbs! SERIOUSLY! That's enough to put you in a diabetic coma. Fancy coffees can be a milkshake "in drag". Be wary of what you order.

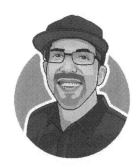

Bill spent ten years in the U.S. Army where drinking a cup of coffee was all about caffeine, not taste. Bill was shocked to discover the extreme varieties of specialty drinks! There are more choices at Starbucks alone than any other restaurant in this book. In case you are coffee naïve, like Bill, he has added a brief explanation of what these fancy drinks might include throughout the chapter.

Disclaimer:

The following information is a culmination of information from the Starbucks website as well as other published sources. It represents our best efforts to be clear and accurate. Surprisingly, Starbucks, as a company, makes it very hard to get the nutrition information about their products. Yes, they have a nutrition information search engine on their website, but it is slow, prone to crashing and difficult to use.

We have made every effort to provide accurate information but occasionally, estimates were made when exact information could not be found. For example, how many carbs are in the Starbucks bread or tortillas? This data is not published. Additionally, since Starbucks sources their bread rolls and tortillas from multiple subcontractors depending on store location, there will be inconsistencies in the nutritional make-up from each source. Lastly, in the interest of simplicity, carb counts were rounded to the nearest whole number.

I was surprised to learn that some Starbucks drinks are only available is certain sizes (i.e. iced drinks do not come in the "short" size) which explains why each drink is not reflected in every size category (Short, Tall, Venti, Grande, etc.).

Friends, we know you love your coffee, so bear with us regarding the shocking news that is about to be unveiled. We award Starbucks a giant sad face because we do not feel they are "transparent" enough with their nutritional information.

STARBUCKS: 10 CARBS OR LESS

DRINKS

ADD ONS

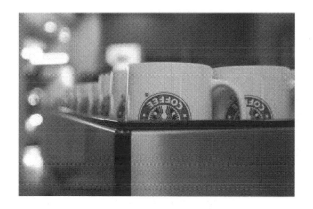

Almond Milk
1g carbs Short
1g carbs Tall
1g carbs Grande
2g carbs Venti

Coconut Milk
1g carbs Short
2g carbs Tall
2g carbs Grande
3g carbs Venti

Non-Fat Milk
1g carbs Short

2g carbs Tall
3g carbs Grande
5g carbs Venti

Whole Milk
1g carbs Short
2g carbs Tall
3g carbs Grande
5g carbs Venti

2% Milk
1g carbs Short
2g carbs Tall
3g carbs Grande
5g carbs Venti

Soy Milk
2g carbs Short
3g carbs Tall
4g carbs Grande
7g carbs Venti

Extras (per serving)
2g carbs Caramel Drizzle
1g carbs Espresso Shot
0g carbs Flavored Sugar Free Syrup, one pump (choices are:
vanilla, caramel, cinnamon dolce, hazelnut and peppermint
(seasonal))
5g carbs Flavored Syrup, one pump
6g carbs Matcha Green Tea Powder, one scoop
1g carbs Mocha Drizzle
7g carbs Mocha Syrup
1g carbs Protein & Fiber Powder, one scoop
2g carbs Tall Whipped Cream for Cold Drinks
3g carbs Grande Whipped Cream for Cold Drinks
3g carbs Venti Whipped Cream for Cold Drinks
1g carbs Short Whipped Cream for Hot Drinks
2g carbs Tall Whipped Cream for Hot Drinks
2g carbs Grande Whipped Cream for Hot Drinks
2g carbs Venti Whipped Cream for Hot Drinks

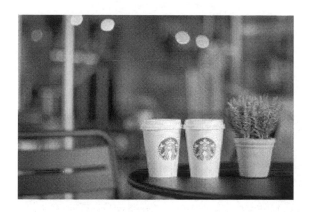

Hot Espresso (All unsweetened unless noted)

Espresso
An espresso is basically really, really strong coffee, served in a teeny, tiny, cup.
1g carbs Solo Espresso
2g carbs Doppio (Double) Espresso
3g carbs Triple Espresso
4g carbs Quad (4 shots) Espresso
2g carbs Solo Espresso Con Panna
3g carbs Doppio Espresso Con Panna
4g carbs Triple Espresso Con Panna
5g carbs Quad Espresso Con Panna
2g carbs Solo Espresso Macchiato with Whole Milk
3g carbs Doppio Espresso Macchiato with Whole Milk
5g carbs Triple Espresso Macchiato with Whole Milk
7g carbs Quad Espresso Macchiato with Whole Milk

Caffé Americano
Caffé Americano is an espresso served in a regular cup with added hot water.
2g carbs Short Caffé Americano, 2 pumps of sugar-free vanilla syrup
3g carbs Tall Caffé Americano
3g carbs Grande Starbucks Blonde Caffé Americano

3g carbs Grande Caffé Americano
4g carbs Venti Caffé Americano

Caffé Latte
Fancy presentation that contains a shot of espresso, lots of steamed milk, and foam on top.
7g carbs Short Caffé Latte with 2% Milk
8g carbs Short Starbucks Blonde Vanilla Latte with Almond Milk
10g carbs Short Vanilla Bean Coconut Milk Latte
9g carbs Short Latte Macchiato with 2% Milk
9g carbs Short Latte Macchiato with Whole Milk
4g carbs Short Starbucks Blonde Caffé Latte with Almond Milk
4g carbs Short Caffé Latte with Almond Milk
6g carbs Tall Caffé Latte with Almond Milk
7g carbs Short Caffé Latte with Coconut Milk
10g carbs Short Caffé Latte with Nonfat Milk
9g carbs Short Caffé Latte with Whole Milk

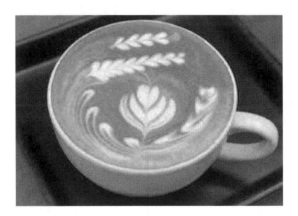

Cappuccino
Drink contains equal amounts of espresso, steamed milk, and milk foam.
8g carbs Short Cappuccino with 2% Milk
9g carbs Tall Cappuccino with 2% Milk
4g carbs Short Starbucks Blonde Cappuccino with Almond Milk
6g carbs Short Cappuccino with Almond Milk
6g carbs Tall Cappuccino with Almond Milk

6g carbs Tall Starbucks Blonde Cappuccino with Almond Milk
7g carbs Grande Cappuccino with Almond Milk
10g carbs Venti Cappuccino with Almond Milk
7g carbs Short Cappuccino with Coconut Milk
8g carbs Short Cappuccino with Nonfat Milk
9g carbs Tall Cappuccino with Nonfat Milk
8g carbs Short Cappuccino with Soy Milk
8g carbs Short Cappuccino with Whole Milk
9g carbs Tall Cappuccino with Whole Milk

Cordusio
An espresso enhanced mocha (extra shot of espresso, whole milk, mocha)
9g carbs Short Cordusio with Almond Milk

Flat White
Made with a shot of espresso and steamed milk, and no foam on top.
4g carbs Short Starbucks Blonde Flat White with Almond Milk
2g carbs Short Flat White, ½ Almond Milk & ½ water steamed
5g carbs Short Flat White with Almond Milk
6g carbs Tall Flat White with Almond Milk
6g carbs Tall Starbucks Blonde Flat White with Almond Milk
7g carbs Grande Flat White with Almond Milk
7g carbs Grande Starbucks Blonde Flat White with Almond Milk
9g carbs Venti Flat White with Almond Milk
7g carbs Short Flat White with Coconut Milk
9g carbs Short Flat White with Whole Milk

Skinny Mocha
Espresso, steamed milk and chocolate
10g carbs Short Skinny Mocha with skinny sugar-free Mocha Sauce

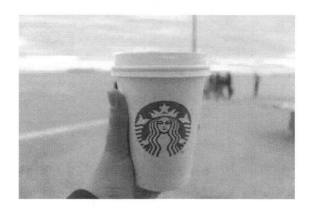

HOT BREWED COFFEE (ALL UNSWEETENED UNLESS NOTED)

Blonde Roast
Light bodied flavor that is soft and mellow.
0g carbs Venti Blonde Roast
0g carbs Short Blonde Roast
0g carbs Tall Blonde Roast
0g carbs Grande Blonde Roast

Caffé Misto
One/One mix of coffee and steamed milk aka café au lait
5g carbs Short Caffé Misto with 2% Milk
8g carbs Tall Caffé Misto with 2% Milk
10g carbs Grande Caffé Misto with 2% Milk
4g carbs Short Caffé Misto with Almond Milk
5g carbs Tall Caffé Misto with Almond Milk
7g carbs Grande Caffé Misto with Almond Milk
7g carbs Venti Caffé Misto with Almond Milk
4g carbs Short Caffé Misto with Coconut Milk
6g carbs Tall Caffé Misto with Coconut Milk
7g carbs Grande Caffé Misto with Coconut Milk
7g carbs Venti Caffé Misto with Coconut Milk
5g carbs Short Caffé Misto with Nonfat Milk
8g carbs Tall Caffé Misto with Nonfat Milk

10g carbs Grande Caffé Misto with Nonfat Milk
6g carbs Short Caffé Misto with Soy Milk
10g carbs Tall Caffé Misto with Soy Milk
5g carbs Short Caffé Misto with Whole Milk
8g carbs Tall Caffé Misto with Whole Milk
10g carbs Grande Caffé Misto with Whole Milk

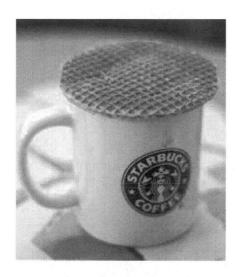

Clover® Brewed Coffee
Personalized coffee brewed with clover technology.
0g carbs Short Clover® Brewed Coffee
0g carbs Tall Clover® Brewed Coffee
0g carbs Grande Clover® Brewed Coffee
0g carbs Venti Clover® Brewed Coffee

Pike Place® Roast
Popular blend that meets a wide range of tastes.
0g carbs Short Pike Place® Roast
0g carbs Tall Pike Place® Roast
0g carbs Grande Pike Place® Roast
0g carbs Venti Pike Place® Roast

Decaf Pike Place® Roast
Popular decaf blend that meets a wide range of tastes.

0g carbs Short Decaf Pike Place® Roast
0g carbs Tall Decaf Pike Place® Roast
0g carbs Grande Decaf Pike Place® Roast
0g carbs Venti Decaf Pike Place® Roast

Featured Dark Roast

Full-bodied, bold, robust flavor.
0g carbs Short Featured Dark Roast
0g carbs Tall Featured Dark Roast
0g carbs Grande Featured Dark Roast
0g carbs Venti Featured Dark Roast

FRAPPUCCINO® BEVERAGES

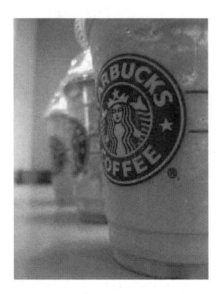

Iced, blended coffee made with a coffee or crème base and usually topped with whipped cream and sauces. Basically, it's a coffee milkshake. PASS!

> *Would you believe there are NO Frappuccino® beverages to share in DIRTY, LAZY, KETO Fast Food Guide: 10 Carbs or Less. NOT ONE! All are too high in carbs! The lowest carb Frappuccino on the Starbucks menu is 30g carbs for a "Tall Crystal Ball Frappuccino® with Almond Milk".*

ICED ESPRESSO (ALL UNSWEETENED UNLESS NOTED)

Iced Caffé Americano
Diluted espresso with hot water served over ice.
2g carbs Tall Iced Caffé Americano
3g carbs Grande Iced Caffé Americano
4g carbs Venti Iced Caffé Americano
3g carbs Grande Iced Starbucks Blonde Caffé Americano

Doubleshot on Ice
Shots of espresso over ice, shaken with your selected dairy added at the end.
4g carbs Tall Doubleshot on Ice with 2% Milk
5g carbs Grande Doubleshot on Ice with 2% Milk
8g carbs Venti Doubleshot on Ice with 2% Milk
3g carbs Tall Doubleshot on Ice with Almond Milk
3g carbs Grande Doubleshot on Ice with Almond Milk
6g carbs Venti Doubleshot on Ice with Almond Milk
4g carbs Tall Doubleshot on Ice with Coconut Milk
4g carbs Grande Doubleshot on Ice with Coconut Milk
7g carbs Venti Doubleshot on Ice with Coconut Milk
5g carbs Tall Doubleshot on Ice with Nonfat Milk
5g carbs Grande Doubleshot on Ice with Nonfat Milk
8g carbs Venti Doubleshot on Ice with Nonfat Milk
5g carbs Tall Doubleshot on Ice with Soy Milk
6g carbs Grande Doubleshot on Ice with Soy Milk
10g carbs Venti Doubleshot on Ice with Soy Milk
4g carbs Tall Doubleshot on Ice with Whole Milk

5g carbs Grande Doubleshot on Ice with Whole Milk
8g carbs Venti Doubleshot on Ice with Whole Milk

Iced Caffé Latte
Espresso plus cold milk poured over ice.
4g carbs Tall Iced Caffé Latte with Almond Milk
5g carbs Grande Iced Caffé Latte with Almond Milk
7g carbs Venti Iced Caffé Latte with Almond Milk
7g carbs Tall Iced Caffé Latte with Coconut Milk
10g carbs Grande Iced Caffé Latte with Coconut Milk
10g carbs Tall Iced Caffé Latte with Nonfat Milk
10g carbs Tall Iced Caffé Latte with Whole Milk

Cold Foam Cappuccino
Iced espresso under a frothed cold foam.
9g carbs Grande Iced Starbucks Blonde Cold Foam Cappuccino
9g carbs Grande Iced Cold Foam Cappuccino

Iced Skinny Espresso
Espresso over ice with Nonfat Milk and often sugar-free syrup.
9g carbs Tall Iced Skinny Cinnamon Dolce Latte with Nonfat Milk
10g carbs Tall Iced Skinny Mocha with Nonfat milk
8g carbs Grande Iced Skinny Mocha

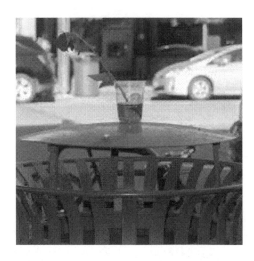

ICED BREWED COFFEE (ALL UNSWEETENED UNLESS NOTED)

Cold Brew
Ground whole bean that you let steep in cold water for 20 hours for a mild, sweet flavor without acidity.
0g carbs Tall Nariño 70 Cold Brew
0g carbs Grande Nariño 70 Cold Brew
0g carbs Venti Nariño 70 Cold Brew
0g carbs Trenta Nariño 70 Cold Brew
1g carbs Tall Starbucks Cold Brew Coffee with Almond Milk

Iced Coffee
Coffee over ice.
0g carbs Tall Iced Coffee
0g carbs Grande Iced Coffee
0g carbs Venti Iced Coffee
0g carbs Trenta Iced Coffee
1g carbs Tall Iced Coffee with Almond Milk
3g carbs Grande Iced Coffee with 2% milk
2g carbs Grande Iced Coffee with Coconut Milk
1g carbs Tall Iced coffee, 2 pumps of Sugar Free Cinnamon Dolce Syrup
8g carbs Grande Starbucks Low Calorie Iced Coffee + Milk

Foam Brew
Cold brew coffee topped with cold foam.
4g carbs Tall Cold Foam Cold Brew
5g carbs Grande Cold Foam Cold Brew

Nitro Cold Brew
Cold brew infused with nitrogen.
0g carbs Grande Nitro Cold Brew
4g carbs Tall Nitro Cold Brew with Sweet Cream

Coconut Cold Brew
Brewed coffee over ice with a float of coconut milk.
9g carbs Tall Toasted Coconut Cold Brew with 2% Milk

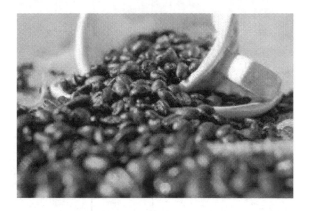

8g carbs Tall Toasted Coconut Cold Brew with Almond Milk
10g carbs Grande Toasted Coconut Cold Brew with Almond Milk
8g carbs Tall Toasted Coconut Cold Brew with Coconut Milk
9g carbs Tall Toasted Coconut Cold Brew with Nonfat Milk
9g carbs Tall Toasted Coconut Cold Brew with Soy Milk
9g carbs Tall Toasted Coconut Cold Brew with Whole Milk

HOT TEA (ALL UNSWEETENED UNLESS NOTED)

0g carbs Royal English Breakfast Tea (all sizes)
0g carbs Comfort Wellness Brewed Tea (all sizes)
0g carbs Teavana® Organic Chai Tea (all sizes)
0g carbs Emperor's Cloud and Mist® Green Tea (all sizes)
0g carbs Jade Citrus Mint Green Tea (all sizes)
0g carbs Organic Jade Citrus Mint™ Brewed Tea (all sizes)
0g carbs Mint Majesty™ Herbal Tea (all sizes)
0g carbs Passion Tango™ Herbal Tea (all sizes)
0g carbs Peach Tranquility® Herbal Tea (all sizes)
0g carbs Rev Up Wellness Brewed Tea (all sizes)
0g carbs Teavana® Earl Grey Brewed Tea (all sizes)
0g carbs Youthberry® White Tea (all sizes)
2g carbs Short Defense Wellness Brewed Tea
2g carbs Tall Defense Wellness Brewed Tea
3g carbs Grande Defense Wellness Brewed Tea
3g carbs Venti Defense Wellness Brewed Tea

4g carbs Short Chai Tea Latte, 2 pumps of sugar-free Cinnamon Dolce

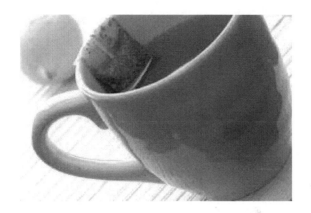

ICED TEA (ALL UNSWEETENED UNLESS NOTED)

Shaken Iced Black Tea
0g carbs Tall Teavana® Shaken Iced Black Tea
2g carbs Tall Teavana® Shaken Iced Black Tea with Coconut Milk
8g carbs Tall Teavana® Shaken Iced Black Tea, Lightly Sweetened (with sugar)

Shaken Iced Green Tea
0g carbs Tall Teavana® Shaken Iced Green Tea
2g carbs Tall Teavana® Shaken Iced Green Tea with Coconut Milk
8g carbs Tall Teavana® Shaken Iced Green Tea, Lightly Sweetened (with sugar)

Shaken Iced Passion Tango Tea
0g carbs Tall Teavana® Shaken Iced Passion Tango™ Tea
2g carbs Tall Teavana® Shaken Iced Passion Tango™ Tea with Coconut Milk
8g carbs Tall Teavana® Shaken Iced Passion Tango™ Tea, Lightly Sweetened (with sugar)

Shaken Peach Citrus White Tea

0g carbs Tall Teavana® Shaken Peach Citrus White Tea Infusion
2g carbs Tall Teavana® Shaken Peach Citrus White Tea Infusion
with Coconut Milk
8g carbs Tall Teavana® Shaken Peach Citrus White Tea Infusion,
Lightly Sweetened (with sugar)

Shaken Pineapple Black Tea

0g carbs Tall Teavana® Shaken Pineapple Black Tea Infusion,
2g carbs Tall Teavana® Shaken Pineapple Black Tea Infusion with
Coconut Milk
8g carbs Tall Teavana® Shaken Pineapple Black Tea Infusion,
Lightly Sweetened (with sugar)

Shaken Strawberry Green Tea

0g carbs Tall Teavana® Shaken Strawberry Green Tea Infusion,
2g carbs Tall Teavana® Shaken Strawberry Green Tea Infusion
with Coconut Milk
8g carbs Tall Teavana® Shaken Strawberry Green Tea Infusion,
Lightly Sweetened (with sugar)

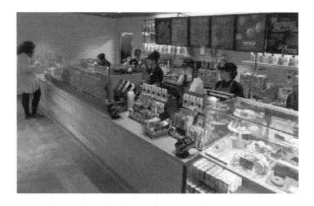

FOOD AT STARBUCKS

BREAKFAST FOOD

5g carbs Sausage, Cheddar & Egg Breakfast Sandwich, no bread
3g carbs Bacon, Gouda & Egg Breakfast Sandwich, no bread
5g carbs Double-Smoked Bacon, Cheddar & Egg Sandwich, no bread
4g carbs Carved Ham & Swiss Breakfast Sandwich, no bread
2g carbs Egg & Cheddar Breakfast Sandwich, no bread
2g carbs Ham & Cheese Croissant, no bread
4g carbs Red.-Fat Turkey Bacon & Cage Free Egg White Breakfast Sandwich, no bread
3g carbs Slow-Roasted Ham, Swiss & Egg Breakfast Sandwich, no bread
5g carbs Spicy Chorizo, Monterey Jack & Egg Breakfast Sandwich, no bread
5g carbs Spinach, Feta & Cage Free Egg White Breakfast Wrap, no wrap
5g carbs Seared Steak, Egg & Tomatillo Wrap, no tortilla
9g carbs Chicken Chorizo Tortilla Sous Vide Egg Bites, no tortilla strips
9g carbs Sous Vide Egg Bites: Bacon & Gruyere

LUNCH SANDWICHES

5g carbs Chicken & Double-Smoked Bacon Sandwich, No bread
6g carbs Turkey & Havarti Sandwich, no bread
5g carbs Chicken Caprese sandwich, no bread
4g carbs Chicken BLT Salad Sandwich, no bread
3g carbs Egg Salad Sandwich, no bread
3g carbs Italian-Style Ham & Spicy Salami Sandwich, no bread
4g carbs Roasted Tomato & Mozzarella Panini, no bread
6g carbs Turkey and Pastrami Rueben, no bread

SALADS

4g carbs Cauliflower Tabbouleh Side Salad, no vinaigrette

7g carbs Garden Greens & Shaved Parmesan Side Salad, no dressing

https://www.starbucks.com/menu/catalog/nutrition?drink=all#view_control=nutrition

DUNKIN' DONUTS: HACKS FROM THE AUTHORS OF DIRTY, LAZY, KETO

When we were visiting NYC to run the New York City Marathon, Stephanie was floored by how many Dunkin' Donuts (or excuse me, "Dunkin'") stores were available. She couldn't walk one city block without smelling those freshly made donuts! Stephanie is sure they have great coffee here, but seriously, how can you avoid buying a donut? Because she knows her self-control isn't strong enough to actually walk inside a Dunkin' Donuts, Stephanie prefers to use the drive thru (if available). Then she is able to order exactly what she wants without succumbing to carbolicious urges! (In the interest of full disclosure, Stephanie ate at least a dozen of those stupid donuts in NYC - UGH!)

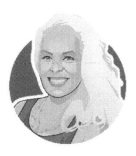

> *Here is a true story about my first time ordering a sugar-free iced coffee at DD. It tasted SO GOOD that I was worried they gave me a drink with REAL sugar. I actually got back in line at the drive thru just so I could ask the cashier if indeed, my drink was sugar free. Yes, I'm that kind of obsessive about my DIRTY, LAZY, KETO diet!*

Bill loves the coffee at Dunkin' Donuts because they offer a variety of sugar-free flavors that can be added to your coffee:

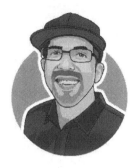

French Vanilla
Hazelnut
Toasted Almond
Blueberry
Raspberry
Coconut - All Sugar Free!

Bill also likes the variety of breakfast items. It's not often that a fast food restaurant offers such a variety of eggs and meat to include veggie egg whites, turkey sausage, and even Angus Steak. Lunch food options are very limited. If you came to a Dunkin' Donuts for a sandwich or wrap, you better be prepared to eat a breakfast item.

Note to Reader: The dairy products used by Dunkin' Donuts are different from those used at Starbucks. Do not assume all coffee houses use the same ingredients! For example, the almond milk option at Dunkin' Donuts is HIGHER in carbs than traditional dairy additives here which suggests they are using a "sweetened" Almond Milk.

All of the Dunkin' Donuts coffee "Flavored Shots" are sugar-free (French Vanilla, Hazelnut, Toasted Almond etc.) whereas the "Flavored Swirls" are not sugar-free (Mocha Swirl, Hazelnut Swirl) so this makes ordering simpler. The Flavored Shots do have one or two carbs depending on size so this may be due to the sugar alcohols in the mix. Depending on your opinions about sugar alcohols, some keto followers choose to subtract those carb grams from net carb count.

DUNKIN' DONUTS: 10 CARBS OR LESS

DRINKS

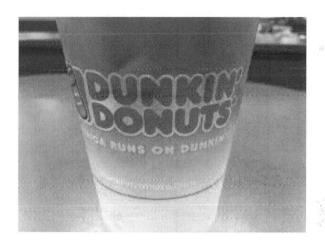

ADD ONS

Almond Milk
3g carbs Small
5g carbs Medium
6g carbs Large
9g carbs Extra Large

Skim Milk
2g carbs Small
3g carbs Medium
3g carbs Large

4g carbs Extra Large

Whole Milk
1g carbs Small
2g carbs Medium
3g carbs Large
4g carbs Extra Large

Cream
1g carbs Small
2g carbs Medium
2g carbs Large
3g carbs Extra Large

All Sugar Free Flavored Syrups
(French Vanilla, Hazelnut, Toasted Almond, Blueberry, Raspberry, Coconut)
1g carbs Small
1g carbs Medium
2g carbs Large

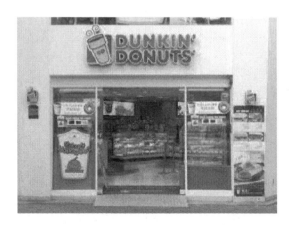

Hot Coffee- Unsweetened unless noted

Americano
Espresso served in a regular cup with added hot water.
1g carbs Small Americano
2g carbs Medium Americano
2g carbs Large Americano

Cappuccino
Drink contains equal amounts of espresso, steamed milk, and milk foam.
7g carbs Small Hot Cappuccino, Whole Milk
10g carbs Medium Hot Cappuccino, Whole Milk

Latte
Fancy presentation that contains a shot of espresso, lots of steamed milk, and foam on top.
10g carbs Small Latte with Whole Milk
10g carbs Small Latte with Skim Milk

Espresso
An espresso is basically really, really strong coffee, served in a teeny, tiny, cup.
1g carbs Single Shot Espresso
7g carbs Single Shot Espresso with Sugar

French Vanilla
Flavored Dunkin Donuts brewed coffee.
1g carbs Small French Vanilla Hot Coffee
1g carbs Medium French Vanilla Hot Coffee
2g carbs Large French Vanilla Hot Coffee

Hot Coffee
1g carbs Small Hot Coffee
1g carbs Medium Hot Coffee
2g carbs Large Hot Coffee
2g carbs Extra Large Hot Coffee
3g carbs Small Hot Coffee with Almond Milk
6g carbs Medium Hot Coffee with Almond Milk
8g carbs Large Hot Coffee with Almond Milk

10g carbs Extra Large Hot Coffee with Almond Milk
4g carbs Small Hot Coffee with Cream
5g carbs Medium Hot Coffee with Cream
7g carbs Large Hot Coffee with Cream
5g carbs Extra Large Hot Coffee with Cream
2g carbs Small Hot Coffee with Milk
3g carbs Medium Hot Coffee with Milk
5g carbs Large Hot Coffee with Milk
6g carbs Extra Large Hot Coffee with Milk
3g carbs Small Hot Coffee with Skim Milk
4g carbs Medium Hot Coffee with Skim Milk
5g carbs Large Hot Coffee with Skim Milk
6g carbs Extra Large Hot Coffee with Skim Milk
2g carbs Small Hot Coffee with Splenda® No Calorie Sweetener
3g carbs Medium Hot Coffee with Splenda® No Calorie Sweetener
5g carbs Large Hot Coffee with Splenda® No Calorie Sweetener
6g carbs Extra Large Hot Coffee with Splenda® No Calorie
Sweetener
3g carbs Small Hot Coffee with Skim Milk and Splenda® No Calorie
Sweetener
5g carbs Medium Hot Coffee with Skim Milk and Splenda® No
Calorie Sweetener
8g carbs Large Hot Coffee with Skim Milk and Splenda® No Calorie
Sweetener
10g carbs Extra Large Hot Coffee with Skim Milk and Splenda® No
Calorie Sweetener

Hot Macchiato
Steamed milk goes in first, followed by the espresso then milk foam making pretty layers.
7g carbs Small Hot Macchiato with Whole Milk
8g carbs Small Hot Macchiato with Skim Milk

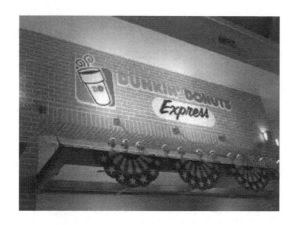

ICED COFFEE- UNSWEETENED UNLESS NOTED

2g carbs Small Iced Coffee
2g carbs Medium Iced Coffee
3g carbs Large Iced Coffee
4g carbs Small Iced Coffee with Almond Milk
7g carbs Medium Iced Coffee with Almond Milk
9g carbs Large Iced Coffee with Almond Milk
3g carbs Small Iced Coffee with Cream
4g carbs Medium Iced Coffee with Cream
5g carbs Large Iced Coffee with Cream
3g carbs Small Iced Coffee with Milk
5g carbs Medium Iced Coffee with Milk
6g carbs Large Iced Coffee with Milk
3g carbs Small Iced Coffee with Skim Milk
5g carbs Medium Iced Coffee with Skim Milk
6g carbs Large Iced Coffee with Skim Milk
5g carbs Small Iced Coffee with Skim Milk and Splenda® No
Calorie Sweetener
7g carbs Medium Iced Coffee with Skim Milk and Splenda® No
Calorie Sweetener
10g carbs Large Iced Coffee with Skim Milk and Splenda® No
Calorie Sweetener
4g carbs Small Iced Coffee with Splenda® No Calorie Sweetener
5g carbs Medium Iced Coffee with Splenda® No Calorie Sweetener
7g carbs Large Iced Coffee with Splenda® No Calorie Sweetener

Iced Latte
Espresso plus cold milk poured over ice.
10g carbs Small Iced Latte with Whole Milk
10g carbs Small Iced Latte with Skim Milk

Iced Macchiato
Steamed milk goes in first, followed by the espresso then milk foam making pretty layers over ice.
8g carbs Small Iced Macchiato with Skim Milk
7g carbs Small Iced Macchiato with Whole Milk

Cold Brew Coffee
2g carbs Small Cold Brew Coffee
2g carbs Medium Cold Brew Coffee
3g carbs Large Cold Brew Coffee
2g carbs Small Cold Brew Coffee with Cream
4g carbs Medium Cold Brew Coffee with Cream
6g carbs Large Cold Brew Coffee with Cream

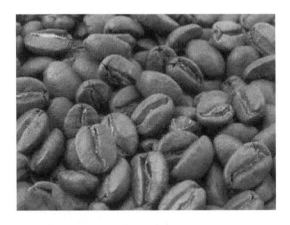

Hot Tea- Unsweetened unless noted
0g carbs Small Bold Breakfast Black Tea
0g carbs Medium Bold Breakfast Black Tea
0g carbs Large Bold Breakfast Black Tea

0g carbs Small Chamomile Fields Herbal Infusion

0g carbs Medium Chamomile Fields Herbal Infusion
0g carbs Large Chamomile Fields Herbal Infusion

0g carbs Small Cool Mint Herbal Infusion
0g carbs Medium Cool Mint Herbal Infusion
0g carbs Large Cool Mint Herbal Infusion

0g carbs Small Decaf Breakfast Black Tea
0g carbs Medium Decaf Breakfast Black Tea
0g carbs Large Decaf Breakfast Black Tea

0g carbs Small Harmony Leaf Green Tea
0g carbs Medium Harmony Leaf Green Tea
0g carbs Large Harmony Leaf Green Tea

0g carbs Small Hibiscus Kiss Herbal Infusion
0g carbs Medium Hibiscus Kiss Herbal Infusion
0g carbs Large Hibiscus Kiss Herbal Infusion

Iced Tea- Unsweetened unless noted

1g carbs Small Iced Green Tea
2g carbs Medium Iced Green Tea
2g carbs Large Iced Green Tea

1g carbs Small Iced Tea
2g carbs Medium Iced Tea
2g carbs Large Iced Tea

3g carbs Small Iced Tea Blueberry Flavored Tea
4g carbs Medium Iced Tea Blueberry Flavored Tea
6g carbs Large Iced Tea Blueberry Flavored Tea

3g carbs Small Iced Tea Raspberry Flavored
4g carbs Medium Iced Tea Raspberry Flavored
6g carbs Large Iced Tea Raspberry Flavored

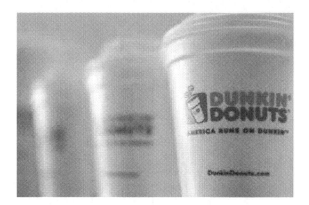

FOOD

Breakfast

9g carbs Kosher Veggie Bacon and Veggie Sausage Croissant Sandwich, no bread
9g carbs Kosher Veggie Bacon and Veggie Sausage Wake-Up Wrap, no wrap

3g carbs Bacon, Egg & Cheese Wake-Up Wrap, no wrap
3g carbs Bacon, Egg & Cheese on Croissant, no bread
3g carbs Bacon, Egg & Cheese on English Muffin, no bread
3g carbs Bacon, Egg & Cheese on a Plain Bagel, no bread
5g carbs Double Sausage Breakfast Sandwich, no bread
2g carbs Egg & Cheese Wake-Up Wrap, no wrap
2g carbs Egg & Cheese on Croissant, no bread
2g carbs Egg & Cheese on English Muffin, no bread
2g carbs Egg & Cheese on a Plain Bagel, no bread
3g carbs Ham, Egg & Cheese Wake-Up Wrap, no wrap
3g carbs Ham, Egg & Cheese on Croissant, no bread
3g carbs Ham, Egg & Cheese on English Muffin, no bread
3g carbs Ham, Egg & Cheese on a Plain Bagel, no bread
2g carbs Sausage, Egg & Cheese Wake-Up Wrap, no wrap
2g carbs Sausage, Egg & Cheese on Croissant, no bread
2g carbs Sausage, Egg & Cheese on English Muffin, no bread
2g carbs Sausage, Egg & Cheese on a Plain Bagel, no bread
3g carbs Turkey Sausage Sandwich on English Muffin, no bread

3g carbs Turkey Sausage Wake Up Wrap, no wrap
1g carbs Veggie Egg White Sandwich on an English Muffin, no bread
1g carbs Veggie Egg White Wake-Up Wrap, no wrap

LUNCH

3g carbs Big N' Toasted, no bread
7g carbs Chicken Croissant Sandwich, no bread
2g carbs Turkey Sausage Flatbread, no bread
3g carbs Angus Steak Egg & Cheese, no bread
3g carbs Turkey Bacon & Cheddar Ciabatta, no bread, extra cheese

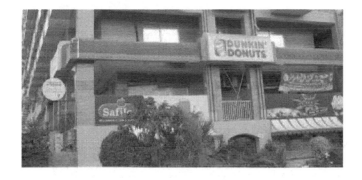

DESSERTS

7g carbs Cinnamon Munchkin
9g carbs Glazed Blueberry Munchkin
8g carbs Glazed Chocolate Munchkin
7g carbs Glazed Munchkin
9g carbs Glazed Old Fashioned Munchkin
9g carbs Jelly Munchkin
6g carbs Old Fashioned Munchkin
7g carbs Powdered Munchkin

https://www.dunkindonuts.com/content/dam/dd/pdf/nutrition.pdf

McDonald's McCafé: Hacks from the Authors of Dirty, Lazy, Keto

Stephanie recommends the medium Sugar-Free French Vanilla Iced Coffee when you're in the mood for a splurge. It feels decadent, like

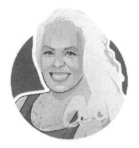

enjoying a fancy dessert. If you are like her, and love the McCafé Chocolate Chip Frappé, try making this alternative at home with this simple low carb recipe: ice, cream, coffee, unsweetened cocoa powder, Splenda, some protein powder – blend - then add a palmful of sugar-free chocolate chips. Voila!

Bill's hack is to use the McDonald's app on your smart phone where freebies and discounts are regularly offered. Everyone in your party can download the app and purchase their food separately to enjoy free and discounted promotional items!

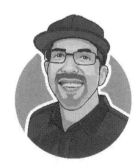

Another cost saving hack is to order your black coffee with a second large cup of ice. You can make your own iced coffee for a third of the cost.

Note to Reader from Bill:

Figuring out the carb count for the McDonald's McCafé menu proved to be very difficult! Depending on the source, I found varying numbers for many of the drinks and even the add ons for dairy and flavored syrup. The following is the result of my extensive knowledge as well as placing my confidence in certain respected sources for nutritional content.

The McDonald's provided nutrition calculator is not very helpful. The low carb choices for add ons are not available in most cases, which makes finding low carb options is that much harder. The Sugar Free French Vanilla Syrup is only listed as on option for a few of the coffees in the nutrition calculator, but in reality, it is offered in any of the drinks where a syrup is allowed. Can you believe that in the McDonald's nutrition calculator under "Iced French Vanilla Latte", you do not have the option to choose the Sugar Free French Vanilla Syrup, just the regular French Vanilla Syrup? Crazy, right? It is listed as an option for the "Iced Latte" and that is how I was able to determine the carb count.

The below choices are listed as they are on the menu for the most part and the contents are the typical contents unless specified. For example, the Latte and Iced Latte come with whole milk typically at McDonald's so I would not list that as the dairy for these drinks.

You might be surprised to learn that DIRTY, LAZY, KETO has awarded a sad face to McDonald's McCafé due to their cumbersome online nutritional information. We expect more from the nation's largest fast food restaurant that serves more than a billion cups of coffee each year! [2]

When placing your order, be specific about the ingredients you would like. Don't be embarrassed to ask for what you need. You are paying for this food or drink, so it should be prepared per your instructions.

When in doubt, check the printed label on the side of the cup. "SF" denotes sugar free, for example.

---

[2] https://www.factretriever.com/mcdonalds-food-facts

McDonald's McCafé: 10 Carbs or Less

ADD ONS

4g carbs Small Whole Milk
6g carbs Medium Whole Milk
8g carbs Large Whole Milk

5g carbs Small Non-Fat Milk
7g carbs Medium Non-Fat Milk
9g carbs Large Non-Fat Milk

2g carbs Small Light Cream
3g carbs Medium Light Cream
5g carbs Large Light Cream

** Full Cream is an option but is not covered on the McDonald's
website **

6g carbs Small Sugar Free French Vanilla Syrup
7g carbs Medium Sugar Free French Vanilla Syrup

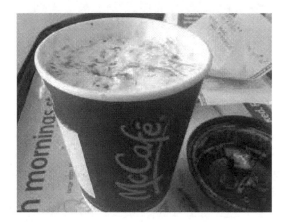

COFFEE-UNSWEETENED UNLESS NOTED

Hot Brewed Coffee
1g carbs Small Hot Coffee
2g carbs Medium Hot Coffee
2g carbs Large Hot Coffee

Hot Espresso
0g carbs Small Espresso Americano Coffee
0g carbs Medium Espresso Americano Coffee
1g carbs Large Espresso Americano Coffee

Cappuccino
5g carbs Small Cappuccino, substitute whole cream for milk
7g carbs Medium Cappuccino, substitute whole cream for milk
9g carbs Large Cappuccino, substitute whole cream for milk
4g carbs Small Cappuccino, ½ whole milk ½ steamed water
6g carbs Medium Cappuccino, ½ whole milk ½ steamed water
9g carbs Large Cappuccino, ½ whole milk ½ steamed water
7g carbs Small Cappuccino with Nonfat Milk

French Vanilla Latte

7g carbs Small Sugar Free French Vanilla Latte, substitute full cream, light SF French Vanilla Syrup

Carmel Macchiato

4g carbs Small Caramel Macchiato, no caramel syrup, no milk
4g carbs Medium Caramel Macchiato, no caramel syrup, no milk
5g carbs Large Caramel Macchiato, no caramel syrup, no milk

Iced Coffee

6g carbs Small Iced Coffee with Sugar Free French Vanilla Syrup, no dairy
8g carbs Medium Iced Coffee with Sugar Free French Vanilla Syrup, no dairy
5g carbs Small Sugar Free French Vanilla Iced Coffee, substitute full cream
7g carbs Medium Sugar Free Vanilla Iced Coffee, with cream

2g carbs Small Cold Brewed Coffee
2g carbs Medium Cold Brewed Coffee
3g carbs Large Cold Brewed Coffee

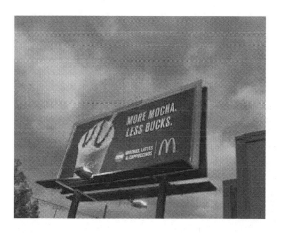

Iced Latte

4g carbs Small Iced Latte with Light Cream
6g carbs Medium Iced Latte with Light Cream

7g carbs Small Iced Nonfat Latte
9g carbs Medium Iced Nonfat Latte
6g carbs Small Iced Latte with Whole Milk
8g carbs Medium Iced Latte with Whole Milk
10g carbs Large Iced Latte with Whole Milk

Iced Carmel Macchiato
4g carbs Small Iced Caramel Macchiato, no caramel syrup, no milk
4g carbs Medium Iced Caramel Macchiato, no caramel syrup, no milk
4g carbs Large Iced Caramel Macchiato, no caramel syrup, no milk

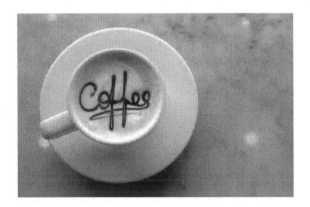

https://www.mcdonalds.com/us/en-us/about-our-food/nutrition-calculator.html

2. BURGERS

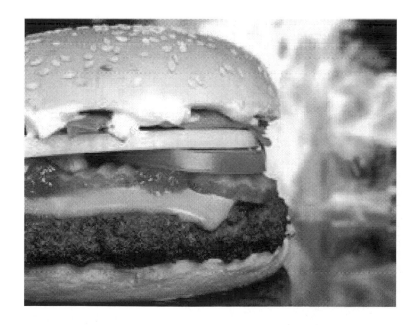

BURGER HACKS FROM DIRTY, LAZY, KETO:

No matter what burger chain you choose, try the following keto hacks to reduce the carbs in your meal. These are general tips to think about.

*The authors were shocked to learn that protein at fast food burger chains often contain substantial carbs. This might be due to the meat being mixed with fillers, like oats. Apparently, a hamburger isn't just a hamburger when you are eating out! The chicken is not innocent either. Poultry is sometimes prepared in a brine of sugar and salt water.

*Throw away the bun! Go topless and bottomless – heyyyyy! (that joke never gets old, people).

*Ask the burger chain to "wrap" your hamburger using lettuce leaves, instead of the bun. Some might throw a sad little piece of lettuce next to your burger, but many chains are used to this request and will go all-out to wrap that beauty.

*Chop up your hamburger and add it to a purchased salad.

*If the restaurant has a "topping bar", create a little salad with the complimentary toppings and top with your burger.

*Keto friendly toppings include mustard, mayonnaise, pickles, cheese, jalapeños, avocado, ranch dressing, bacon, guacamole, sour cream and butter.

*Avoid sugar-laden sauces like ketchup, "special sauce", and barbeque sauce.

*Ketchup is a hidden danger. I have seen carb counts as high as 8g carbs for a single packet! Always specify "no ketchup" so you don't end up having to scrape ketchup off of your burger.

*If you're really getting nitpicky, avoid tomatoes and onions for their small carb contribution.

*Grilled is better than fried.

*Order breakfast anytime. Eggs are keto-fabulous!

*Is there a salad bar? That's a terrific alternative.

*Throw away any croutons served on top of your salad right away.

*Enjoy water from the soda fountain – (that weird little gray bar that is super small.)

*Keep an eye on seasonal or regional offerings for surprises. For example, in Hawaii SPAM is served at breakfast.

*Ask for extra, extra, extra lettuce on your burger and create a free salad!

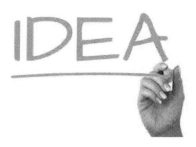

McDonald's: Hacks from the Authors of DIRTY, LAZY, KETO

Stephanie suggests ordering off of the "dollar" or "value" menu to get more food for less money. This Value Menu changes frequently, but, at the time of this

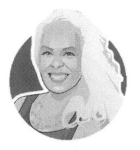

publication, here is a suggestion: Order the dollar menu "McDouble" (no ketchup) and add "special sauce" with lettuce instead of the bun. This tastes pretty much the same as a Big Mac®, but without the price tag!

Want eggs? Um, yes please! Now that McDonald's serves breakfast all day long, ordering

eggs is easy. But you want real eggs, right? Be sure to request the "round eggs" so you will in fact receive a real egg, and not the powdered stuff!

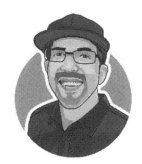

Want a free Quarter Pounder? Bill suggests calling the number listed on the bottom of your receipt to take a quick survey. Afterward, McDonald's will provide you with a code to redeem for a BOGO free sandwich at the register. FREE!

In case you skimmed over the McDonald's McCafé section, Bill would also like to remind you about the McDonald's free app for your smart phone, where freebies and promotion items are updated weekly.

Lastly, just because you hear "You Deserve A Break Today" from this famous chain doesn't give you license to indulge. Be aware of marketing and its effect on your ordering.

McDonald's: 10 Carbs or Less

BREAKFAST

2g carbs Double Order of Scrambled Eggs (1 egg each) (Not on the menu)
5g carbs Turkey Sausage Scramble Bowl
2g carbs Egg McMuffin, no bread
2g carbs Sausage McMuffin, no bread
4g carbs Two Sausage Burritos, no tortillas
0g carbs Butter

Drinks

0g carbs Half and Half, single container
1g carbs Unsweetened Coffee

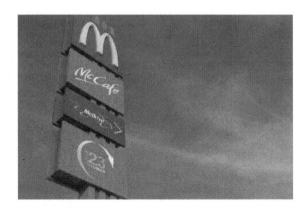

LUNCH & DINNER

7g carbs "Bunless" Big Mac
5g carbs Quarter Pounder with cheese, no bread
5g carbs Cheeseburger without bun or substitute lettuce for buns
4g carbs McDouble without bun or ketchup

2g carbs Grilled Chicken Sandwich, without bun or substitute lettuce for buns

Salads
6g carbs Premium Bacon Ranch Salad with Grilled Chicken (w/o dressing)
10g carbs Premium Caesar Salad with Grilled Chicken (w/o dressing)
2g carbs Side Salad
4g carbs Newman's Own Low-Fat Balsamic Vinaigrette
7g carbs Newman's Own Ranch

Drinks
0g carbs Diet Coke®
0g carbs Iced Tea
1g carbs Unsweetened Coffee

https://www.mcdonalds.com/us/en-us/about-our-food/nutrition-calculator.html

BURGER KING: HACKS FROM THE AUTHORS OF DIRTY, LAZY, KETO

Stephanie reminds you that when ordering a "customized burger" at Burger King, you are getting a freshly cooked hamburger, not one that has been possibly sitting around. That's awesome!

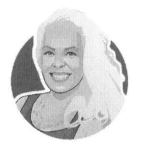

While waiting for your order, be aware of how many times you visit the soda bar for refills. If you are choosing the Minute Maid Light Lemonade, those refills can add up the carbs fast and furiously!

Bill spent his youth flipping burgers at BK. He worked on a military base where literally HUNDREDS of soldiers would blow through his drive-thru window at lunch demanding "HOT WHOPPAS!"

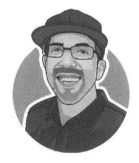

Bill's tips to keep the carbs low at the second largest fast food chain in the world include: ordering a garden salad, removing croutons, and then adding your hamburger or grilled chicken all chopped up on top of your salad.

In terms of salad dressing, do not choose the fat-free which is loaded with 18 grams of sugar.

Instead, choose Ken's Ranch (2 grams of carbs) or Ken's Golden Italian (4 grams of carbs).

BURGER KING: 10 CARBS OR LESS

BREAKFAST
3g carbs Fully Loaded Croissan'wich, no bread
1g carbs Sausage Egg and Cheese, no bread
5g carbs Double Sausage and Egg Breakfast Platter
2g carbs Eggnormous Burrito in a Bowl, no hash browns, no tortilla

Drinks
0g carbs Large BK Joe Coffee, Unsweetened

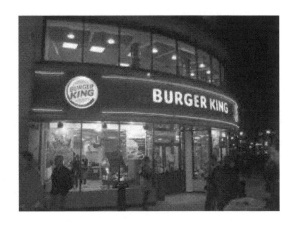

LUNCH & DINNER
3g carbs Whopper with Cheese, no bread, no ketchup
1g carbs Sourdough King Single, plain with no bread
2g carbs two Double Cheeseburgers, plain with no bread
1g carbs Grilled Chicken Sandwich, no bread
8g carbs Grilled Chicken Club Sandwich, no bread
3g carbs Tendergrill Chicken Sandwich, no bread
10g carbs 4-piece Chicken Nugget's

Salad
2g carbs Garden Side Salad
8g carbs Tendergrill Chicken Garden Salad, no Dressing, no croutons
2g carbs Ken's Ranch Dressing
4g carbs Ken's Golden Italian

Drinks
0g carbs Diet Coke®
4g carbs Large Minute Maid® Light Lemonade
0g carbs Unsweetened Iced Tea

https://www.bk.com/pdfs/nutrition.pdf

WENDY'S: HACKS FROM THE AUTHORS OF **DIRTY, LAZY, KETO**

Stephanie worked her first fast food job at Wendy's. At the ripe age of 15, she was in charge of stocking the salad bar. Bring back the

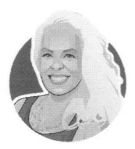

salad bar, Wendy's! That was keto heaven. Nowadays, Stephanie suggests ordering burgers from the value meal, cutting them up, and adding them to your side salad. The same can be done for grilled chicken, of course. If you are feeling "spendy", try ordering an extra chicken filet for your sandwich. Wendy's will also add extra bacon and cheese upon request.

Want eggs? Bill says you can order real eggs at Wendy's. They don't open until late morning, though, so don't come here for an early breakfast.

Be wary of the fancy salads at Wendy's as most are filled with carbolicious additives. You are better off with a simple side salad and grilled meats.

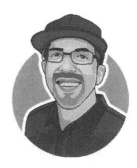

WENDY'S: 10 CARBS OR LESS

BREAKFAST
No breakfast served at most locations.

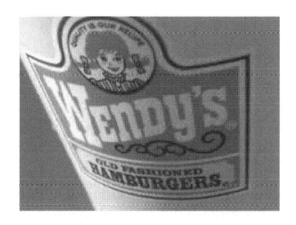

LUNCH/DINNER
3g carbs Grilled Chicken Breast, no sauce, no bread
0g carbs Single Hamburger, no sauce, no bread
2g carbs Applewood Bacon Smoked Burger, no bread, no sauce
3g carbs Triple Baconator, plain with no bread

Salads
5g carbs Garden Side Salad, no dressing or croutons
4g carbs Caesar Side Salad, no dressing or croutons
2g carbs Lemon Garlic Caesar Dressing
2g carbs Ranch Dressing

Drinks
0g carbs Coffee any size

0g carbs single container of Half and Half
0g carbs Diet Coke®
0g carbs Unsweetened Iced Tea
4g carbs Large Minute Maid Light Lemonade®

https://menu.wendys.com/en_US/categories/?_ga=2.24900346.159
5443625.1539549824-693296166.1539549824

DAIRY QUEEN: HACKS FROM THE AUTHORS OF DIRTY, LAZY, KETO

Stephanie has such fond memories of walking to DQ for a dipped cone in the hot summers of her childhood, that going there as an adult for a healthy lunch might trigger a craving for soft serve. These associations are hard to overcome! Pass.

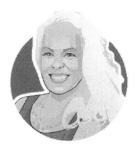

Bill is impressed with the variety of low carb options here, especially in the salad arena. They offer enough choices to keep keto life

interesting! Additionally, like In-N-Out Burger, the DQ cashiers are accustomed to folks ordering double and triple burgers.

Since Bill likes spicy food, his favorite DQ menu item is the Flamethrower (jalapeño flavor!) burger without the bun at 4 grams of carbs.

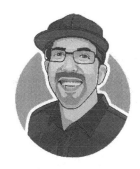

DAIRY QUEEN: 10 CARBS OR LESS

BREAKFAST
No Breakfast Served

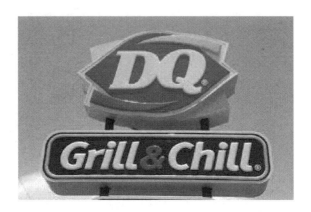

LUNCH/DINNER
4g carbs Flamethrower Grill Burger (sauce included), no bread
4g carbs Grilled Chicken Sandwich, no bread
5g carbs Turkey BLT, no bread, no sauce
2g carbs DQ Ultimate Burger, no bread
3g carbs Original Cheeseburger, no bread, no sauce
5g carbs Grilled Chicken Bacon Ranch, no bread

Salads
9g carbs Grilled Chicken BLT Salad (1 ranch dressing included)

3g carbs Side Salad, no dressing
2g carbs Marzetti Buttermilk Ranch Dressing
2g carbs Marzetti Creamy Caesar Dressing
2g carbs Marzetti Light Italian Dressing

Drinks
0g carbs Diet Coke®
0g carbs Sprite Zero®

https://www.dairyqueen.com/us-en/Company/Nutrition/Food-Treats/?localechange=1&

IN-N-OUT: HACKS FROM THE AUTHORS OF DIRTY, LAZY, KETO

Stephanie suggests going somewhere else since they don't have salads or chicken. Why no other options? Such limited choices. Thumbs down. Wah!

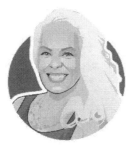

Bill loves going to In-N-Out. He likes that the staff is familiar with ordering "protein style" which means having the burger wrapped in lettuce instead of a bun.

Feeling brave? Try ordering off the secret menu (not listed on the signage):

Double/Double – two burger patties (with or without cheese)

3X3 – three burger patties (with or without cheese)

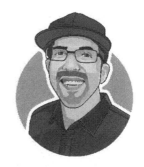

4x4 – four burger patties (with or without cheese)

"Animal Style" – mustard cooked burger

"The Flying Dutchman" – two slices of American cheese between two burger patties

IN-N-OUT: 10 CARBS OR LESS

BREAKFAST
No Breakfast Offered

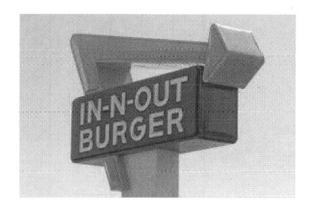

LUNCH/DINNER
8g carbs Hamburger "protein style", lettuce wrapped
3g carbs Hamburger "protein style", lettuce wrapped, no onion, no spread
8g carbs Cheeseburger "protein style", lettuce wrapped
4g carbs Cheeseburger "protein style", lettuce wrapped, no onion, no spread
8g carbs Double Double "protein style" lettuce wrapped
4g carbs Double Double "protein style" lettuce wrapped, no onion, no spread
8g carbs Hamburger "animal style", no bread (mustard cooked burger)
4g carbs Hamburger "animal style", no bread (mustard cooked burger), no spread
2g carbs The Flying Dutchman (2 Burger Patties, 2 slices American Cheese ONLY)

Drinks
0g carbs Diet Coke®
4g carbs Large Minute Maid Light Lemonade®
0g carbs Iced Tea, Unsweetened
0g carbs Hot Coffee

http://www.in-n-out.com/nutrition.aspx

JACK IN THE BOX: HACKS FROM THE AUTHORS OF DIRTY, LAZY, KETO

Stephanie loved ordering the turkey burger from Jack in the Box. What happened to that on the menu? Dang it.

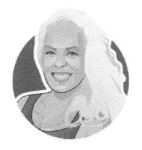

When ordering your sandwich, ask for "extra lettuce" when you say "no bread". How much did that cost? If the cashier is being kind to you, keep adding sides of lettuce. For just pennies you might be able to put together a salad here with all those sides!

Bill suggests ordering off the Jr. menu to save money and enjoy more protein. The value menu Jr. Bacon Cheeseburgers, without bread, really hit the spot.

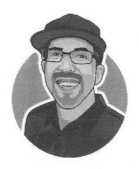

JACK IN THE BOX: 10 CARBS OR LESS

BREAKFAST
4g carbs Loaded Breakfast Sandwich, no bread
1g carbs Meat Lovers Breakfast Burrito, no tortilla
1g carbs Extreme Sausage Sandwich, no bread
2g carbs Steak and Egg Breakfast Burrito, no hash browns, no tortilla
3g carbs Grande Sausage Breakfast Burrito, no hash browns, no tortilla

Drinks
1g carbs Regular Decaf Premium Roast Coffee, unsweetened
2g carbs Large Decaf Premium Roast Coffee, unsweetened
1g carbs Regular Premium Roast Coffee, unsweetened
2g carbs Large Premium Roast Coffee, unsweetened

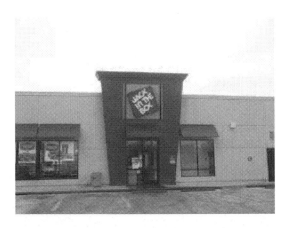

LUNCH/DINNER
5g carbs 4 Piece Grilled Chicken Strips

2g carbs Jr. Jack, no bread
3g carbs Jr. Jack with Cheese, no bread
3g carbs Jr. Bacon Cheeseburger, no bread
0g carbs Bacon and Swiss Buttery Jack, no bread
1g carbs Ultimate Cheeseburger, lettuce wrapped, no ketchup
2g carbs Double Jack, no bread
3g carbs Sourdough Grilled Chicken Club, no bread
2g carbs Chicken Fajita Pita, no salsa, no pita

Salads
10g carbs Grilled Chicken Salad, no Dressing, no croutons
8g carbs Chicken Club Salad with Grilled Chicken, no dressing, no croutons
3g carbs Bacon Ranch Dressing
2g carbs Light Ranch Dressing
3g carbs Low Fat Vinaigrette

Drinks
0g carbs Diet Coke®
0g carbs Diet Dr. Pepper®
2g carbs Large Gold Peak Fresh Brewed Iced Tea, Unsweetened

http://static.jackinthebox.com/pdfs/nutritional_brochure.pdf

Carl's Jr./Hardee's: Hacks from the Authors of DIRTY, LAZY, KETO

Stephanie suggests adding bacon or guacamole to your meal for added fat.

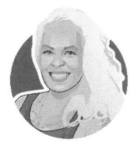

Bill says Carl's Jr./Hardee's totally rocks the low carb "hustle". They even have the words "low carb" on their menu! How cool is that? The Thickburgers are hearty and filling, and you won't feel weird ordering special requests as the burger is already

wrapped in lettuce. No explanations necessary!

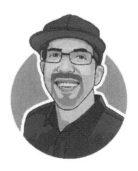

We are awarding Carl's Jr./Hardee's a gold star for directly including and acknowleding us low carb eaters on your menu. You make us feel special and loved.

CARL'S JR./HARDEE'S: 10 CARBS OR LESS

BREAKFAST
8g carbs Low Carb Breakfast Bowl
1g carbs Steak and Egg Breakfast Burrito, no tortilla
2g carbs Loaded Breakfast Burrito, no tortilla, no hash browns
2g carbs The Breakfast Burger, no bread, no hash browns
4g carbs Monster Biscuit, no bread
2g carbs Sausage Egg and Cheese Biscuit, no bread
6g carbs Grilled Cheese Breakfast Sandwich with Ham, no bread

Drinks
0g carbs Large Black Coffee

LUNCH/DINNER

5g carbs Low Carb Super Star with Cheese, lettuce wrapped
6g carbs Low Carb 1/3-pound Thickburger, lettuce wrapped
8g carbs Low Carb 1/2-pound Thickburger, lettuce wrapped
4g carbs Famous Star Burger, no bread
3g carbs Double Cheeseburger, no bread
7g carbs Low Carb Charbroiled Chicken Club, lettuce wrapped
8g carbs Kids Hand Breaded Chicken Tenders (2 pcs)

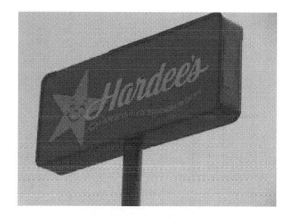

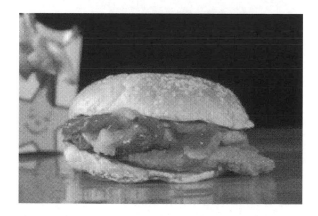

Salads
7g carbs Charbroiled Chicken Salad, no croutons, no onion, no dressing
5g carbs Side Salad, no croutons, no dressing

Drinks
0g carbs Diet Coke®
4g carbs Large Minute Maid Light Lemonade®
0g carbs Diet Dr. Pepper®
0g carbs Large Gold Peak unsweetened iced tea

https://www.carlsjr.com/nutrition

FIVE GUYS: HACKS FROM THE AUTHORS OF DIRTY, LAZY, KETO

Stephanie suggests the Cheese Veggie Sandwich (wrapped in lettuce of course) as a fun alternative to eating burgers. Ask for extra veggies!

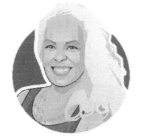

Interesting Fact: FIVE GUYS KETO SECRET - When you order a Bacon Cheeseburger, you can add extra cheese and bacon for FREE. Please note that this is ONLY for the Bacon Cheeseburger, otherwise you will be charged!

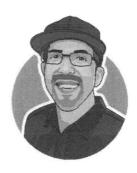

Lastly, we would like to recognize Five Guys with a DIRTY, LAZY, KETO GOLD STAR for their keto-friendly menu and easy to use nutritional guide! It's rare to find a fast food restaurant that "fesses up" to the carb count of their buns, so that fact alone sets them apart. You are able to "build your own" sandwich by choosing individual protein and toppings with an accurate carb count from their website. Thanks, Five Guys. Gold start to you!

FIVE GUYS: 10 CARBS OR LESS

BREAKFAST
No Breakfast Served

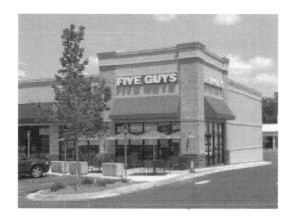

LUNCH/DINNER
Meat
0g carbs Bacon (2 pieces)
0g carbs Hamburger Patty
2g carbs Hot Dog

Toppings
3g carbs A.1® Sauce
0g carbs Cheese (1 slice)
1g carbs Green Peppers
1g carbs Grilled Mushrooms
0g carbs Hot Sauce
0g carbs Jalapeño Peppers
5g carbs Ketchup

1g carbs Lettuce
0g carbs Mayonnaise
0g carbs Mustard
2g carbs Onions / Grilled Onions
1g carbs Pickles
2g carbs Relish
2g carbs Tomatoes

6g carbs Cheese Veggie Sandwich, no bread, regular toppings

Drinks
0g carbs Diet Coke®
0g carbs Diet Sprite®

http://www.fiveguys.com/-/media/Public-
Site/Files/FiveGuysNutrition_Aug2014_CAN_E.ashx

WHATABURGER: HACKS FROM THE AUTHORS OF DIRTY, LAZY, KETO

Stephanie suggests ordering extra Jalapeño Creamy Ranch Dressing as it goes with just about everything on the menu and tastes sooooo good!

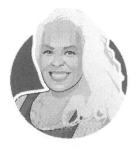

Bill suggests trying to order "scrambled eggs and bacon" a la carte to save money and not waste food by throwing buns away. More and more fast food restaurants are honoring these types of special requests. Bill is often surprised at how helpful the cashiers can be if you tell them you need a

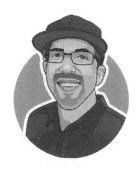

"diabetic" friendly meal. (Note, Bill didn't lie about being a diabetic. He simply said he wants a "diabetic type of meal". Folks understand diabetes and can be sympathetic to a medical need, but not necessarily helpful about the term keto.

WHATABURGER: 10 CARBS OR LESS

BREAKFAST
0g carbs Sausage Egg and Cheese Sandwich, no bread
3g carbs Sausage, Egg, and Cheese Taquito, no tortilla
3g carbs Scrambled Eggs and Bacon (a la carte)
3g carbs Breakfast On A Bun® with Sausage, no bread
2g carbs Jalapeño Cheddar Biscuit with Sausage, no bread

Drinks-Unsweetened
0g carbs Small Coffee, Colombian
0g carbs Medium Coffee, Colombian
0g carbs Large Coffee, Colombian
1g carbs Small Decaf Coffee, Colombian
2g carbs Medium Decaf Coffee, Colombian
2g carbs Large Decaf Coffee, Colombian

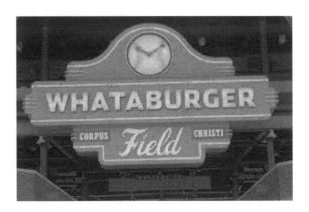

LUNCH/DINNER
2g carbs Whataburger Patty Melt, no bread

5g carbs Double Meat Whataburger with 2 Cheese, Bacon, and Jalapeños, no bread
5g carbs Triple Meat Cheese Whataburger, no bread
5g carbs Monterey Melt, no bread
4g carbs Jalapeño and Cheese Whataburger, no bread
7g carbs Green Chile Double, no bread

4g carbs Chicken Fajita Taco, no tortilla
3g carbs Grilled Chicken Melt plus side of Lettuce, no bread
3g carbs Grilled Chicken Melt, no bread

Salads
2g carbs Garden Salad
5g carbs Garden Salad with Grilled Chicken, no dressing
3g carbs Apple and Cranberry Salad, no dressing, no cranberries
6g carbs Apple and Cranberry Salad with Grilled Chicken, no dressing, no cranberries

Dressing
8g carbs 1000 Island Dressing
0g carbs Balsamic Vinaigrette Dressing
3g carbs Buttermilk Ranch Dressing
2g carbs Jalapeño Ranch Dressing

Drinks
0g carbs Diet Coke®
0g carbs Diet Dr. Pepper®

http://whataburger.com/food/nutrition

3.   MEXICAN

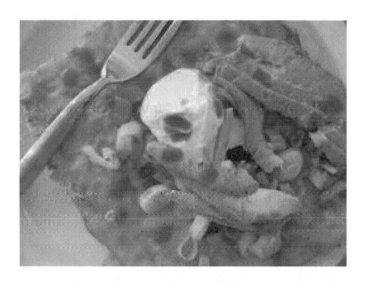

MEXICAN FOOD HACKS FROM THE AUTHORS OF DIRTY, LAZY, KETO

*You can always ask for extra lettuce or extra grilled chicken/steak to make a heartier meal with little or no increase in carbs!

*Avoid chips, shells, beans, rice and tortillas.

*If at a "sit down" restaurant, ask the server to remove the chip basket. Why tempt fate?

*Substitute a bed of lettuce for rice/beans.

*Mexican food keto friendly ingredients: sour cream, cheese, avocado/guacamole, olives and lettuce.

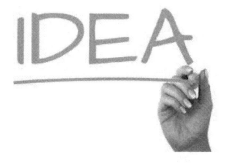

TACO BELL: HACKS FROM THE AUTHORS OF DIRTY, LAZY, KETO

Stephanie suggests ordering "sides" of everything you like: a "side of chicken", "side of lettuce", and a "side of guac" will be cheaper than ordering chicken tacos, eating the insides, and throwing away the tortilla.

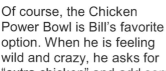

We heard of a funny story about a customer who tried to order a "Nacho Supreme with lettuce instead of chips". It took a few exchanges to get the cashier to understand what she was trying to order. A manager even had to get involved. The cashier couldn't quite comprehend why anyone in their right mind would order nachos without the chips!

Bill says to keep an eye out for seasonal and regional promotional menu items. For example, the "Naked Egg Taco" was a huge hit in our neighborhood.

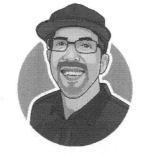

Of course, the Chicken Power Bowl is Bill's favorite option. When he is feeling wild and crazy, he asks for "extra chicken" and add some "Fire Sauce". Bill loves spicy food. The hotter the better! Hot and spicy gives low carb flavor!

Lastly, both authors agreed to award Taco Bell with a DIRTY, LAZY, KETO GOLD STAR for their keto-friendly menu and easy to use nutritional guide!

GOLD STAR! *"TACO BELL CALCULATOR" IS FABULOUS! BE SURE TO USE THIS. THE LINK IS PROVIDED AT THE END OF THIS RESTAURANT SECTION. THEIR LINK EVEN GIVES YOU THE CAPABILITY TO REMOVE THE TORTILLA OR TACO SHELL ETC. FROM YOUR SELECTIONS SO YOU CAN BE EXACT IN YOUR CARB COUNTS. NOT MANY RESTAURANTS DO THIS.*

Taco Bell: 10 Carbs or Less

BREAKFAST

6g carbs Grande Scrambler Burrito with extra eggs, no potatoes, no beans, no tortilla
4g carbs Grilled Breakfast Burrito with extra eggs, no potatoes, to tortilla
3g carbs Mini Skillet Bowl, no potatoes
2g carbs Bacon Breakfast Soft Taco, no shell
2g carbs Sausage Breakfast Quesadilla, no tortilla

Drinks

0g carbs Iced Regular Coffee (one size)
0g carbs Rainforest Coffee (one size)
0g carbs Rainforest Coffee with Nestle® Coffee-Mate™ Sweetened Original Creamer (1 portion creamer)

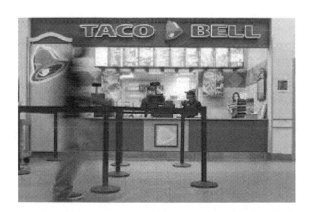

LUNCH/DINNER

Hot Sauce Packets
0g carbs Border Sauce - Diablo
0g carbs Border Sauce - Fire
0g carbs Border Sauce - Hot
0g carbs Border Sauce - Mild
0g carbs Breakfast Salsa

Entrees
10g carbs Crunchy Taco
10g carbs Nacho Cheese Doritos® Locos Taco
10g carbs Fiery Doritos® Locos Taco
10g carbs Cool Ranch® Doritos® Locos Taco
3g carbs Chipotle Chicken Loaded Griller with extra Chicken, no tortilla, no rice or beans
2g carbs Shredded Chicken Burrito with no tortilla, no rice
6g carbs Steak Fresco Burrito Supreme with no beans, no tortilla
7g carbs Beefy 5 Layer Burrito, no tortilla, no refried beans

6g carbs Classic Grilled Chicken Burrito, no tortilla
2g carbs Steak Crunchy Taco with no shell
7g carbs Black Beans (Side)

Power Menu Bowls
5g carbs Chicken Power Menu Bowl, no beans, no rice
7g carbs Chicken Power Menu Bowl with extra Chicken, extra, cheese, extra lettuce, no beans, no rice
7g carbs Steak Power Menu Bowl with Creamy Jalapeño Sauce, no beans, no rice
6g carbs Ground Beef Power Menu Bowl, no beans, no rice

Salads/Nachos
10g carbs Fiesta Taco Salad with Chicken with double extra lettuce, no rice, no beans, no red strip, no shell
7g carbs Fiesta Taco Salad with Chicken with double extra lettuce, no rice, no beans, no red strip, no shell, no fire roasted salsa
8g carbs Fiesta Taco Salad with Steak with double extra lettuce, no rice, no beans, no red strip, no shell, no fire roasted salsa
3g carbs Nachos Supreme with Grilled Chicken, no chips, no nacho cheese sauce
6g carbs Nachos Supreme with Seasoned Beef, no chips, no nacho cheese sauce

4g carbs Nachos Supreme with Grilled Steak, no chips, no nacho cheese sauce

Drinks
0g carbs Diet Pepsi®
0g carbs Diet Dr. Pepper®
0g carbs Diet Mtn. Dew®
0g carbs Aquafina® Sparkling Berry Breeze (Any Size)

https://www.tacobell.com/nutrition/info

DEL TACO: HACKS FROM THE AUTHORS OF DIRTY, LAZY, KETO

Stephanie loves the ground turkey tacos as a great "lean meat alternative". It's unusual to find turkey tacos at a fast food

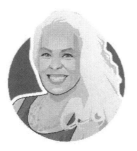

restaurant! Unfortunately, the nutritional information guide for Del Taco doesn't separate the crunchy taco shell or tortilla from what's inside the taco. That being said, when she is feeling spendy, Stephanie loves to order the turkey tacos and just eat what is inside (throwing away the shell or tortilla).

Bill was surprised that the crunchy value taco fit into the DIRTY, LAZY, KETO perimeters of being under ten carbs. Can you believe it? Bill can order a real taco for 7 grams of carbs and it's super cheap. That's a win, win in Bill's playbook!

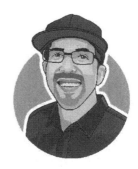

DEL TACO: 10 CARBS OR LESS

BREAKFAST

5g carbs Chorizo Epic Scrambler, no tortilla, no hash brown sticks
5g carbs Epic Scrambler Carne Asada, no tortillas, no hash brown sticks
3g carbs Bacon Breakfast Burrito, no tortilla

Drinks
2g carbs Prima Java Hot Coffee

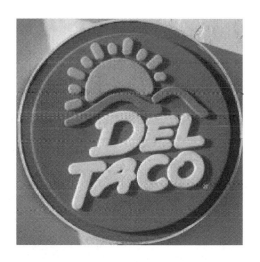

LUNCH/DINNER
6g carbs Mexican Chopped Chicken Salad, no beans, no rice
7g carbs Crunchy Value Taco
1g carbs Crunchy Value Taco, no shell
2g carbs The Del Taco, no shell, extra cheese and lettuce
2g carbs The Turkey Del Taco, no shell, extra cheese and lettuce
4g carbs Classic Grilled Chicken Burrito, no tortilla

5g carbs Del Beef Burrito, no tortilla
4g carbs Original Chicken Roller, no tortilla
5g carbs Double Beef Classic Taco, no shell
2g carbs Mini Cheddar Quesadilla, no tortilla
6g carbs Queso Loaded Nachos with Carne Asada and extra lettuce, No chips and no beans

Burgers
4g carbs Del Cheeseburger, no bread
4g carbs Double Del Cheeseburger with no bread
4g carbs Bacon Double Del Cheeseburger, no bread

Drinks
0g carbs Diet Coke®
4g carbs Large Minute Maid® Light Lemonade
0g carbs Large Gold Peak Tea, unsweetened

https://deltaco.com/files/pdf/nutritionals.pdf

CHIPOTLE: HACKS FROM THE AUTHORS OF DIRTY, LAZY, KETO

Stephanie says Chipotle is the NUMBER ONE fast food restaurant

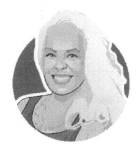

for her diet. She loves to order "double meat" for extra protein. Stephanie suggests ordering extra grilled fajita vegetables (at no extra charge). She is not shy about asking for seconds on other non-meat toppings too –they are happy to keep filling up your bowl! Perfect for a volume eater (so embarrassing).

Bill shares a sneaky tip for getting more protein, but not by increasing the price of your meal. If you ask for the protein to be "split evenly" between two choices, say chicken and steak, you end up getting a ton more meat than if you only ordered one protein.

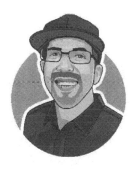

Food for thought here… Bill wonders why Chipotle charges for an extra scoop of protein, but when he says "hold the rice" and/or "hold the beans", he is not receiving a credit on the tab. We know the price of meat is expensive, but come on, guys!

Lastly, we would like to award Chipotle with a DIRTY, LAZY, KETO GOLD STAR for their keto-friendly menu and easy to use nutritional guide! We love you, Chipotle!

CHIPOTLE: 10 CARBS OR LESS

BREAKFAST
No Breakfast Served

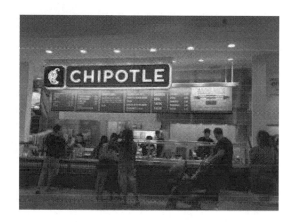

LUNCH/DINNER

Meats/Tofu
0g carbs Chicken
0g carbs Steak
0g carbs Carnitas
1g carbs Barbacoa
1g carbs Chorizo
6g carbs Sofritas (Tofu)

Select Fillings
7g carbs Black Beans, Half Serving
6g carbs Pinto Beans, Half Serving
4g carbs Fajita Vegetables

Select Toppings
4g carbs Queso
2g carbs Fresh Tomato Salsa (Pico de Gallo)
4g carbs Tomatillo-Green Chili Salsa
3g carbs Tomatillo-Red Chili Salsa
1g carbs Sour Cream
1g carbs Cheese
2g carbs Guacamole
1g carbs Romaine Lettuce

Bowls
8g carbs Barbacoa Burrito Bowl (no rice or beans) with extra lettuce, Pico de Gallo salsa, sour cream, cheese and Guacamole
3g carbs Chicken Burrito Bowl (no rice or beans) with extra lettuce, sour cream and cheese
3g carbs Steak Burrito Bowl (no rice or beans) with sour cream, cheese and lettuce

Salads
8g carbs Chicken Salad (no Dressing) with Red Tomatillo Chili Salsa, sour cream, cheese, guac and lettuce
4g carbs Steak Salad with extra Steak (no Dressing) with sour cream, cheese and extra lettuce

Drinks
0g carbs Diet Coke®

https://www.chipotle.com/nutrition-calculator#

EL POLLO LOCO: HACKS FROM THE AUTHORS OF DIRTY, LAZY, KETO

Stephanie likes all the salad options at El Pollo Loco. However, because most of their menu salads contain corn, beans and tomatoes on top, the carb counts of these salads are way over our limit of "10 carbs or less". If you ask the server nicely to omit these offending ingredients, you can broaden your menu selection here.

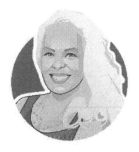

Bill loves El Pollo Loco when he has a coupon. It can get a little pricey here for fast food! If you are a frequent diner at El Pollo Loco, be sure to download their app to get points and earn free rewards. Aside from price, the food here is totally keto friendly. If you focus on the chicken, shrimp, lettuce, cheese, avocado, sour cream, and salsas, you can't go wrong.

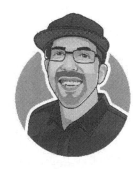

EL POLLO LOCO: 10 CARBS OR LESS

BREAKFAST
No Breakfast Served

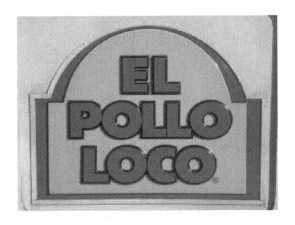

LUNCH/DINNER
0g carbs Flame Grilled Drumstick
0g carbs Flame Grilled thigh
0g carbs Flame Grilled Breast
7g carbs Small Chicken Tortilla Soup w/o tortilla strips
4g carbs Chicken Taco al Carbón, no tortilla
8g carbs Mexican Caesar Bowl, no rice, no tortilla strips, no Dressing
7g carbs Chicken Fajita Burrito, no tortilla, no beans, no rice
4g carbs Side of Broccoli
7g carbs Side of Cole Slaw
3g carbs side of Guacamole

Salads

5g carbs Double Chicken Avocado Salad, no corn, no cotija crumbles, no dressing
5g carbs Classic Chicken Salad, no corn, no tortilla strips, no dressing
6g carbs Loco Side Salad
2g carbs Creamy Cilantro Dressing
2g carbs Ranch Dressing (packet)
3g carbs Lite Creamy Cilantro Dressing (packet)

Salsas

2g carbs House Salsa (Mild)
2g carbs Pico de Gallo (Medium)
2g carbs Avocado Salsa (Hot)
2g carbs Salsa Roja (Fiery)
1g carbs Sour Cream
1g carbs Jalapeño Hot Sauce (packet

Drinks

0g carbs Diet Coke®
0g carbs Diet Dr. Pepper®
0g carbs Gold Peak® Fresh-Brewed Mango Passion Fruit Tea, unsweetened
0g carbs Gold Peak® Fresh-Brewed Unsweetened Iced Tea

https://www.elpolloloco.com/contentAsset/raw-data/865b8079-86ee-4266-8f60-a37c85270ab6/fileAsset/www.fda.gov

107

4.SANDWICHES

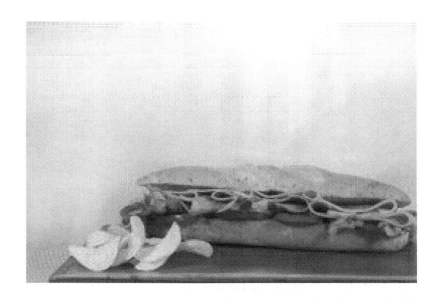

SANDWICH HACKS FROM DIRTY, LAZY, KETO:

*Go topless and bottomless…funny every time! "Hayyyy!" (Yep, I said it again).

*Add extra, extra, extra lettuce to every sandwich order (yes, I said extra three times!).

*Do your research ahead of time and order the lowest carb dressing.

*Ask for dressing on the side.

*Mayo and mustard are preferred keto-fabulous condiments.

*Add avocado to your sandwich to include healthy fats. It's worth the extra money!

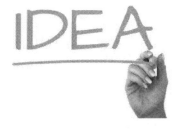

SUBWAY: HACKS FROM THE AUTHORS OF DIRTY, LAZY, KETO

Stephanie suggests ordering the chopped salad. Go crazy with adding the low carb vegetables like pickles, spinach, lettuce, green bell peppers, olives, cheese, banana peppers and jalapeños. Add double meat and cheese, and you will have one filling meal! Her favorite dressing is the spicy chipotle, with extra on the side.

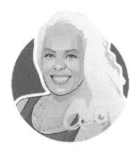

Bill recommends ordering the chopped salad but with tuna fish on top. This is a great

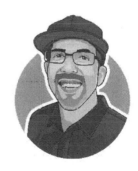

alternative since most restaurants only serve chicken salads.

This salad is totally filling and perfect for big eaters like us!

Subway earns a gold star from DIRTY, LAZY, KETO since they offer an easy to use, interactive nutrition guide on their website. You can enter exactly what toppings are in your order, and learn the precise macros for your meal.

SUBWAY: 10 CARBS OR LESS

BREAKFAST (6 INCH, NO BREAD)
4g carbs Egg and Cheese Omelete sandwich
4g carbs Bacon Egg and Cheese Omelete Sandwich
5g carbs Mega Melt Omelet Sandwich
6g carbs Black Forest Ham, Egg & Cheese Omelete Sandwich
6g carbs Steak, Egg & Cheese Omelete Sandwich
7g carbs Breakfast B.M.T. Omelete Sandwich
5g carbs Sausage, Egg & Cheese Omelete Sandwich
8g carbs Sunrise Subway Melt Omelete Sandwich

Drinks
0g carbs Large Coffee, no sugar

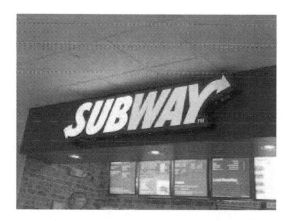

LUNCH/DINNER

Vegetables (6-inch Sub)
0g carbs Banana Peppers

0g carbs Black Olives
1g carbs Cucumbers
0g carbs Green Peppers
0g carbs Jalapeños
1g carbs Lettuce
0g carbs Pickles
1g carbs Red Onions
0g carbs Spinach
1g carbs Tomatoes
3g carbs Avocado
1g carbs Carrots
1g carbs Green Chiles
1g carbs Mushrooms
3g carbs Sweet Peppers

Meats (6-inch Sub)

2g carbs Chicken Patty, Roasted
0g carbs Chicken Strips
5g carbs Chicken Strips, Teriyaki Glazed
2g carbs Cold Cut Combo Meats
3g carbs Egg Patty (regular)
3g carbs Egg Patty (white
2g carbs Ham
2g carbs Italian B.M.T.® Meats
1g carbs Roast Beef
1g carbs Rotisserie-Style Chicken
4g carbs Steak (no cheese)
2g carbs Subway Club® Meats
0g carbs Tuna
2g carbs Turkey Breast
4g carbs BBQ Rib Patty
7g carbs Chicken Enchilada
7g carbs Chicken Salad
1g carbs Chicken Strips, Buffalo Chicken
4g carbs Corned Beef
1g carbs Egg Salad
3g carbs Italian Hero Meats
1g carbs Pastrami
8g carbs Seafood Sensation
1g carbs Sausage, Breakfast
8g carbs Veggie Patty

Cheese (6-inch Sub)
1g carbs American
0g carbs Cheddar
0g carbs Monterey Cheddar
0g carbs Parmesan Cheese
0g carbs Pepper jack
0g carbs Provolone
0g carbs Shredded Mozzarella
0g carbs Swiss

Protein (6-inch Sub)
1g carbs Bacon, 15 grams
3g carbs Guacamole, 35 grams

Sauces and Condiments (6-inch Sub)
1g carbs Bacon (2 strips)
1g carbs Chipotle Southwest Sauce
3g carbs Guacamole
1g carbs Light Mayonnaise (1 T)
0g carbs Mayonnaise (1 T)
1g carbs Mustard, yellow or deli brown (2 tsp.)
0g carbs Oil (1 tsp.)
1g carbs Pepperoni, 3 slices
1g carbs Ranch Dressing
1g carbs Savory Caesar
9g carbs Sweet Onion Sauce, Fat Free
1g carbs Subway® Vinaigrette
0g carbs Vinegar (1 tsp)
9g carbs Barbecue Sauce
1g carbs Buffalo Sauce
4g carbs Creamy Italian
2g carbs Creamy Sriracha
1g carbs Fire Roasted Tomato Sauce
1g carbs Giardiniera
2g carbs Golden Italian
1g carbs Gorgonzola Sauce
7g carbs Honey Mustard Sauce Fat Free
1g carbs Hot Pepper Relish
6g carbs Ketchup
3g carbs Signature Horseradish Sauce
9g carbs Sweet Chili Sauce
2g carbs Sweet Potato Curry

3g carbs Thousand Island Dressing
1g carbs Tzatziki Sauce

Salads (without Dressing)
7g carbs Veggie Delight Salad
6g carbs Double Chicken Chopped Salad
9g carbs Black Forest Ham
9g carbs Oven Roasted Chicken
8g carbs Roast Beef
8g carbs Rotisserie-Style Chicken
9g carbs Subway Club®
9g carbs Turkey Breast
9g carbs Cold Cut Combo
9g carbs Italian B.M.T.®
9g carbs Spicy Italian
9g carbs Steak & Cheese
7g carbs Tuna

Dressings
2g carbs Ranch Dressing
3g carbs Subway Vinaigrette Dressing
0g carbs Oil and Vinegar Dressing
2g carbs Chipotle Southwest

Drinks
0g carbs Diet Coke®
0g carbs Diet Dr. Pepper®

https://www.subway.com/en-us/menunutrition

QUIZNO'S: HACKS FROM THE AUTHORS OF **DIRTY, LAZY, KETO**

Stephanie loves the Chipotle Chicken full sized salad. Who eats half a salad? That's just weird.

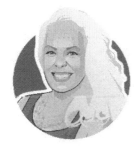

Bill likes the "hot sandwich" option. This keeps things interesting and adds variety. Who doesn't like melted cheese over roast beef?

Bill's favorite is the Spicy Chipotle Pulled Pork Half Salad.

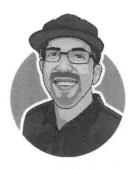

QUIZNO'S: 10 CARBS OR LESS

BREAKFAST

1g carbs Egg and Cheddar Biscuit, no bread
2g carbs Bacon, Egg and Cheddar Biscuit, no bread
2g carbs Steak, Egg and Cheddar Biscuit, no bread
2g carbs Ham, Egg, & Cheddar Biscuit, no bread
1g carbs Sausage, Egg, & Cheddar Biscuit, no bread

0g carbs Large Coffee, unsweetened

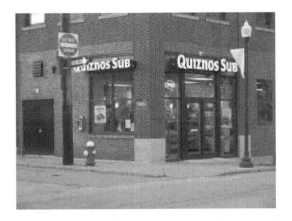

LUNCH/DINNER- NO DRESSING UNLESS SPECIFIED

7g carbs Half Salad Traditional with Red Wine Vinaigrette
9g carbs Half Salad Classic Italian with Red Wine Vinaigrette
8g carbs Half Salad Spicy Monterey with Red Wine Vinaigrette
6g carbs Half Salad Spicy Chipotle Pulled Pork, no onions, no chipotle mayo

5g carbs Half Salad Chipotle Cheddar with Ranch Dressing
5g carbs Half Salad Chipotle Turkey with Ranch Dressing
6g carbs Full Salad Chipotle Turkey with Ranch Dressing
4g carbs Half Salad Ultimate Turkey Club with Ranch with Ranch
Dressing
6g carbs Full Salad Ultimate Turkey Club with Ranch with Ranch
Dressing
5g carbs Half Salad Turkey Bacon Guacamole with Ranch Dressing
4g carbs Full Salad Turkey Ranch and Swiss, no onions, light
tomatoes with Ranch Dressing
6g carbs Half Salad Turkey Ranch & Swiss with Ranch Dressing
8g carbs Full Salad Turkey Ranch & Swiss with Ranch Dressing
8g carbs Half Salad Veggie Guacamole with Ranch Dressing
7g carbs Half Salad Peppercorn Steak
5g carbs Half Salad Chipotle Steak & Cheddar
9g carbs Full Salad Chipotle Steak & Cheddar
7g carbs Side Salad (one Size) with Red Wine Vinaigrette

Chicken
7g carbs Half Salad Chicken Gyro (Limited Time)
10g carbs Full Salad Chicken Gyro (Limited Time)
5g carbs Half Salad Mesquite
7g carbs Full Salad Mesquite
7g carbs Full Salad Southwest Chicken
6g carbs Half Salad Baja
9g carbs Half Salad Carbonara
4g carbs Half Salad Southwest Chicken
7g carbs Full Salad Southwest Chicken

Soups
9g carbs Small Broccoli Cheese
8g carbs Small Chicken Noodle
10g carbs Small Thai Chicken & Rice

Drinks
0g carbs Diet Coke®
0g carbs Diet Mtn. Dew®

http://www.quiznos.com/Libraries/PDFs/NutritionalInfo.sflb.ashx

PANERA BREAD: HACKS FROM THE AUTHORS OF DIRTY, LAZY, KETO

Stephanie says it's hard for her to eat here. The entire place smells like homemade bread and it's too hard to stay on track. The display of sweets as you walk in the door is way too tempting.

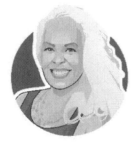

It's like a strip club for carb-addicts. Pass!

Bill was surprised to enjoy his

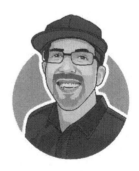

breakfast of Turkey Sausage, Egg White and Spinach Sandwich, no bread with the 0 carb Basil Pesto Sauce. Yum! This was a real treat! Bill's favorite is the Steak & Arugula on Sourdough, no bread. Who can resist tender and succulent steak?

Sadly, we award Panera Bread a sad face as an overall fast food restaurant. They claim to be healthy in their advertising, but upon close examination, DIRTY, LAZY, KETO disagrees. Most of what is on their menu is ridiculously high in carbs. Additionally, it was cumbersome and challenging to get detailed nutritional information from their website.

PANERA BREAD: 10 CARBS OR LESS

BREAKFAST
3g carbs Ham, Egg and Cheese Sandwich, no bread
1g carbs Bacon, Egg and Cheese Sandwich, no bread
2g carbs Turkey Sausage, Egg White and Spinach Sandwich, no bread
3g carbs Sausage, Egg and Cheese Sandwich, no bread
3g carbs Steak, Egg and Cheese Sandwich, no bread

Sauces
0g carbs Basil Pesto Sauce
0g carbs Chipotle Aioli Sauce
2g carbs Sweet Maple

Coffee & Hot Tea
0g carbs Espresso
3g carbs Small Dark Roast Coffee
4g carbs Medium Dark Roast Coffee
5g carbs Large Dark Roast Coffee
2g carbs Small Hazelnut Coffee
3g carbs Medium Hazelnut Coffee
4g carbs Large Hazelnut Coffee
2g carbs Small Light Roast Coffee
3g carbs Medium Light Roast Coffee
4g carbs Large Light Roast Coffee
2g carbs Small Panera Decaf Coffee
2g carbs Medium Panera Decaf Coffee
3g carbs Large Panera Decaf Coffee
0g carbs Hot Teas (all)

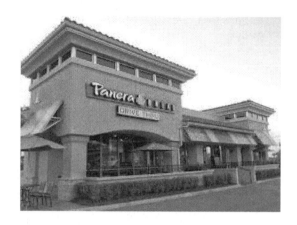

LUNCH/DINNER
10g carbs Steak and Baby Arugula Spinach Sandwich, no bread
6g carbs Steak & Arugula on Sourdough, no bread
2g carbs Roasted Turkey and Avocado BLT, no bread
4g carbs The Italian, no bread
7g carbs Steak and White Cheddar Sandwich, no bread
4g carbs Chicken Chipotle Avocado Melt, no bread

Salads
3g carbs Half Salad Greek Salad, no dressing
7g carbs Full Salad Greek Salad, no dressing
8g carbs Half Salad Green Goddess Cobb Salad with Chicken, no dressing
6g carbs Half Salad Caesar
6g carbs Half Salad Caesar Salad with Chicken, no dressing

Dressings
2g carbs Asian Sesame Vinaigrette Half 1 1/2 Tbsp
4g carbs Asian Sesame Vinaigrette Whole 3 Tbsp
1g carbs Caesar Dressing Whole 1 1/2 Tbsp
2g carbs Caesar Dressing Whole 3 Tbsp
1g carbs Chile Lime Rojo Ranch Half 1 1/2 Tbsp
3g carbs Chile Lime Rojo Ranch Whole 3 Tbsp
0g carbs Greek Dressing Half 1 1/2 Tbsp
1g carbs Greek Dressing Whole 3 Tbsp
1g carbs Green Goddess Dressing Half 1 1/2 Tbsp

3g carbs Green Goddess Dressing Whole 3 Tbsp
4g carbs Low Fat Thai Chili Vinaigrette Half 1 1/2 Tbsp
8g carbs Low Fat Thai Chili Vinaigrette Whole 3 Tbsp
5g carbs Reduced Fat Balsamic Vinaigrette Half 1 1/2 Tbsp
9g carbs Reduced Fat Balsamic Vinaigrette Whole 3 Tbsp
6g carbs White Balsamic Apple Flavored Vinaigrette Half 1 1/2 Tbsp

Iced Drinks and Sodas

0g carbs Medium Plum Ginger Hibiscus Iced Tea
0g carbs Large Plum Ginger Hibiscus Iced Tea
2g carbs Medium Brewed Iced Tea
3g carbs Large Brewed Iced Tea
2g carbs Medium Iced Coffee
4g carbs Large Iced Coffee

0g carbs Diet Pepsi®
0g carbs Diet Mtn. Dew®

https://www.panerabread.com/content/dam/panerabread/documents/nutrition/Panera-Nutrition.pdf

JIMMY JOHN'S: HACKS FROM THE AUTHORS OF DIRTY, LAZY, KETO

Stephanie gets such a kick out of this place! They coined the term "Unwich" (at least to our ears) where a traditional sandwich can be ordered as a lettuce wrap.

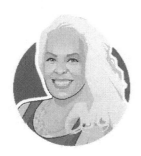

They actually take great pains to wrap it just like a tortilla, so it's easy to eat with one hand. That's pretty convenient! Also, Jimmy John's serves a pickle with your order. That's a terrific alternative to chips, and helps Stephanie get some electrolytes. Yummy!

Bill thinks the sandwich combinations are terrific and creative, although the portion sizes leave much to be desired. He left hungry, wanting to order a second "Unwich". On the plus side, however, Jimmy John's will deliver sandwiches right to your door, even for small orders. How convenient is THAT?

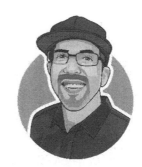

Jimmy John's: 10 Carbs or Less

BREAKFAST
No Breakfast Served

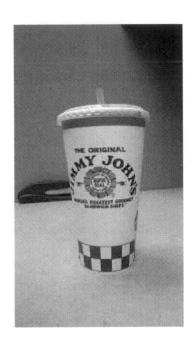

LUNCH/DINNER
4g carbs Italian Night Club Unwich (Lettuce Wrapped)
9g carbs The J.J. Gargantuan Unwich (Lettuce Wrapped)
6g carbs Gourmet Smoked Ham Club Unwich (Lettuce Wrapped)
5g carbs Slim Tuna Salad Unwich & Slim Salami Unwich Combo (Lettuce Wrapped)
1g carbs J.J. B.L.T. Unwich (Lettuce Wrapped)
6g carbs Beach Club Unwich (Lettuce Wrapped)
7g carbs Club Tuna Unwich (Lettuce Wrapped)

Drinks
0g carbs Diet Coke®
0g carbs Sprite Zero®
0g carbs Large Lipton® Iced Tea, unsweetened

https://www.jimmyjohns.com/downloadable-files/NutritionGuide.pdf

JERSEY MIKE'S: HACKS FROM THE AUTHORS OF DIRTY, LAZY, KETO

Stephanie loves the novelty of a "sub in a tub". That's so cute! She feels like she is eating a sandwich, not a salad, by "reframing" it with a new name. This kind of silliness keeps life and the keto diet interesting. Stephanie is a fan!

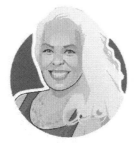

Bill's hack: Any Sub can be ordered in a "tub" as a salad (no bread). Remove the onions and the bell peppers from the "Hot Subs" for the low carb option.

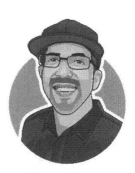

Jersey Mike's: 10 Carbs or Less

BREAKFAST
4g carbs Bacon, Egg and Cheese, no bread
4g carbs Omelet with Ham and Bacon, no bread or wrap
3g carbs Turkey, Egg and Cheese, no bread
4g carbs Steak, Egg and Cheese, no bread

0g carbs Large Coffee, unsweetened

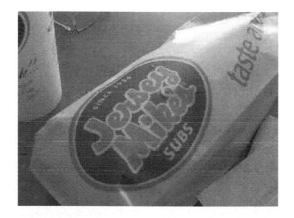

LUNCH/DINNER
0g carbs Grilled Chicken Club in a Tub with extra meat.
5g carbs Chicken Philly Cheese Steak Sub in a Tub, no onions, no sauce
7g carbs Jersey Mike's Famous Philly Sub in a Tub, no onions or peppers
9g carbs Famous Roast Beef and Provolone Sub in a Tub
6g carbs BLT Sub in a Tub
9g carbs "Cancro Special" Sub in a Tub
6g carbs Jersey Shore's Favorite in a Tub
1g carbs Turkey Wrap in a Tub

4g carbs Grilled Veggie Wrap in a Tub

Sides
8g carbs Broccoli Cheese with Florets (cup)
8g carbs Minestrone (cup)

Drinks
0g carbs Diet Pepsi®
0g carbs Diet Mtn. Dew®
0g carbs Large Louisiana Unsweetened Iced Tea

https://www.jerseymikes.com/menu/nutrition

SONIC DRIVE IN: HACKS FROM THE AUTHORS OF DIRTY, LAZY, KETO

Stephanie was surprised about the variety of keto friendly foods on the Sonic menu. Sometimes you just want a change from eating a

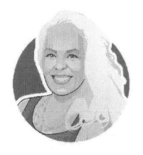

hamburger. With the option of ordering a hot dog or the ability to add chili or Hatch Green Chilis to your meal, the varieties are endless! And what is this Diet Lime Limeade on the menu? Stephanie wants to go there right now just to check that out.

Bill's Hacks:

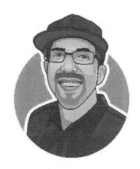

Since ketchup here has 3 carbs, order mustard or mayo instead, (both zero carb condiments).

Order the grilled chicken over the crispy chicken.

Don't forget to have them remove the tater tots from the breakfast burritos (along with the tortilla).

Bill's ultimate favorite has to be that Super SONIC Jalapeño Double Cheeseburger, no bread. LOVE that spicy food, Sonic!

SONIC DRIVE IN: 10 CARBS OR LESS

BREAKFAST

5g carbs Ultimate Meat and Cheese Breakfast Burrito, no tortilla, no potatoes
2g carbs Bacon & Egg Breakfast Toaster, no bread
0g carbs Breakfast Toaster Sausage, no bread
5g carbs Super SONIC Breakfast Burrito, no tortilla, no potatoes
1g carbs Regular 16 oz Coffee, unsweetened

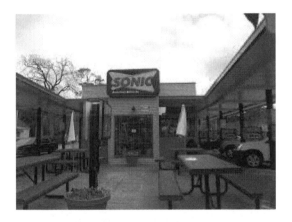

LUNCH/DINNER

6g carbs Super SONIC Bacon Double Cheeseburger, no bread
3g carbs Super SONIC Jalapeño Double Cheeseburger with mustard, no bread
2g carbs Jr Burger, no bread
4g carbs Jr Deluxe Cheeseburger, no bread
3g carbs Jr Double Cheeseburger, no bread

Chicken
4g carbs Grilled Classic Chicken Sandwich, no bread
5g carbs Grilled Chicken Wrap, no tortilla
4g carbs Asiago Caesar Grilled Chicken Club Sandwich, no bread

Hotdogs
8g carbs Footlong ¼ lb. Coney, no bread
8g carbs New York Dog, no bread
3g carbs All Beef Regular Hot Dog, no bread

Toppings
1g carbs American Cheese
1g carbs Avocado
0g carbs Crispy Bacon
1g carbs Grilled Onions
3g carbs Light Ranch Dressing
0g carbs Spicy Jalapeños
1g carbs Chili
0g carbs Hatch Green Chilis

Ultimate Iced Teas-Unsweetened
3g carbs Small Blackberry Diet Green Iced Tea
4g carbs Medium Blackberry Diet Green Iced Tea
6g carbs Large Blackberry Diet Green Iced Tea

1g carbs Small Blackberry Unsweet Iced Tea
2g carbs Medium Blackberry Unsweet Iced Tea
3g carbs Large Blackberry Unsweet Iced Tea

3g carbs Small Diet Green Iced Tea
3g carbs Medium Diet Green Iced Tea
5g carbs Large Diet Green Iced Tea

2g carbs Small Lemon Diet Green Iced Tea
2g carbs Medium Lemon Diet Green Iced Tea
4g carbs Large Lemon Diet Green Iced Tea

3g carbs Small Mango Diet Green Iced Tea
3g carbs Medium Mango Diet Green Iced Tea
6g carbs Large Mango Diet Green Iced Tea

4g carbs Small Minute Maid® Cranberry Diet Green Iced Tea

4g carbs Medium Minute Maid® Cranberry Diet Green Iced Tea
8g carbs Large Minute Maid® Cranberry Diet Green Iced Tea

2g carbs Small Minute Maid® Cranberry Unsweet Iced Tea
4g carbs Medium Minute Maid® Cranberry Unsweet Iced Tea
5g carbs Large Minute Maid® Cranberry Unsweet Iced Tea

1g carbs Small Peach Unsweet Iced Tea
1g carbs Medium Peach Unsweet Iced Tea
2g carbs Large Peach Unsweet Iced Tea

1g carbs Small Raspberry Unsweet Iced Tea
1g carbs Medium Raspberry Unsweet Iced Tea
2g carbs Large Raspberry Unsweet Iced Tea

Signature Limeades
3g carbs Small Diet Cherry Limeade
3g carbs Medium Diet Cherry Limeade
4g carbs Large Diet Cherry Limeade

1g carbs Small Diet Lime Limeade
1g carbs Medium Diet Lime Limeade
1g carbs Large Diet Lime Limeade

Sodas
0g carbs Diet Coke®
0g carbs Diet Dr. Pepper®
0g carbs Sprite Zero®

https://www.sonicdrivein.com/static/pdf/41682-33_NAT_F16_BRO_FA_LR1.pdf

Arby's: Hacks from the Authors of DIRTY, LAZY, KETO

Stephanie suggests asking for sliced lemons and a side of mayo to use as salad dressing. Yes, it might make a mess, but if you squeeze the lemon and a packet of Splenda into the mayo, it makes the most delicious salad dressing!

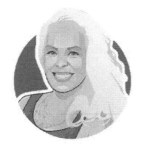

Bill suggests ordering two of the Jalapeño Roast Beef 'n Cheese Sliders (no bread) on a Chopped Side Salad. Since you are tossing the buns, you will save

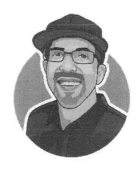

money and actually receive more meat than ordering a regular sized sandwich.

Look at all the things to choose from on the Arby's menu! They have really outdone themselves here, in our opinion.

Lastly, we would like to award Arby's with a DIRTY, LAZY, KETO GOLD STAR for their keto-friendly menu and easy to use nutritional guide!

ARBY'S: 10 CARBS OR LESS

BREAKFAST
No Breakfast Served

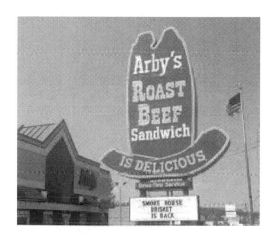

LUNCH/DINNER

Sandwiches
1g carbs Classic Roast Beef, no bread
3g carbs Smokehouse Brisket Sandwich, no bread
4g carbs Bacon Beef and Cheddar Sandwich, no bread, no red ranch
6g carbs Half Pound Beef and Cheddar Sandwich, no bread, no red ranch
3g carbs Classic Beef 'n Cheddar with mayo, no bread, no Arby's Horsey or Red Ranch Sauce
2g carbs French Dip and Swiss Sandwich, no bread, no au jus
6g carbs The Gobbler, no bread, no cranberry spread
5g carbs Cajun Deep-Fried Turkey, no bread, no crispy onions
5g carbs Turkey Avocado Club, no bread, no tomato

5g carbs Turkey Gyro, no bread

Sliders
9g carbs Buffalo Chicken Slider, no bread
9g carbs Chicken 'n Cheese Slider, no bread
2g carbs Ham 'n Cheese Slider, no bread
1g carbs Jalapeño Roast Beef Slider, no bread
2g carbs Pizza Slider, no bread
1g carbs Roast Beef 'n Cheese Slider, no bread
1g carbs Turkey 'n Cheese Slider, no bread

Salads
3g carbs Chopped Side Salad
7g carbs Roast Turkey Farmhouse Salad with Buttermilk Ranch Dressing
8g carbs Roast Turkey Farmhouse Salad Light with Italian Dressing
7g carbs Greek Gyro Salad with Buttermilk Ranch Dressing, no tomatoes

Dressings
2g carbs Light Italian Dressing
8g carbs Dijon Honey Mustard
4g carbs Balsamic Vinaigrette
2g carbs Buttermilk Ranch Dressing

Drinks
0g carbs Diet Coke®
4g carbs Large Minute Maid Light Lemonade®

https://arbys.com/build-a-meal

JAMBA JUICE: HACKS FROM THE AUTHORS OF DIRTY, LAZY, KETO

Stephanie loves smoothies, but this place makes eating low-carb a challenge. Most of the drinks are high in sugar. Yes, the sugars come from fruit, but the reaction the body has to drinking high carb smoothies is no different from eating a candy bar.

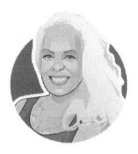

Stephanie does like the fact that Jamba offers "mix ins" like chia seeds, which she tries to eat every day, but the rest of the menu is disappointing. If you are dead set on eating here, then order a "child size" Jamba Juice to reduce your carbs, "make it light", and ask for as many "healthy switches" as the cashier can handle.

Bill's Hacks:

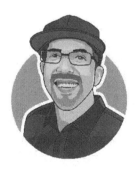

Instead of trying to order a blended Jamba Juice, Bill recommends ordering a Jamba Juice "shot". It's not as fun as a shot of tequila, but it's a lot healthier than these Jamba Juice milkshakes "in drag".

Don't bother trying to get anything to drink here except water, OKAY? There are just WAY too many carbs. If you have to pass through the door, then order a breakfast sandwich. Those will work but only if you remove the bread. THAT'S IT! They don't even sell black coffee here.

We are so disappointed in the overall menu at Jamba Juice that we are awarding this restaurant the DIRTY, LAZY, KETO sad face. Don't let the decorative grass and healthy décor fool you. These smoothies are milkshakes in drag.

JAMBA JUICE: 10 CARBS OR LESS

BREAKFAST
2g carbs Turkey Sausage, Roasted Red Pepper & Gouda Breakfast Sandwich, no bread
2g carbs Spinach 'n Cheese Breakfast Wrap, no wrap
3g carbs Bacon, Roasted Tomato & Spinach Breakfast Sandwich, no bread
2g carbs Turkey Sausage 'n Cheese Breakfast Wrap, no wrap

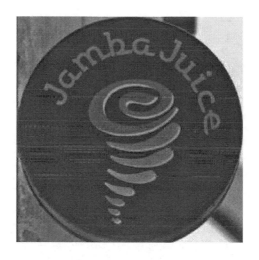

LUNCH
1g carbs Four Cheese Flatbread, no bread
3g carbs Sweet 'n Spicy Chicken Flatbread, no bread and beans

Shots
6g carbs Ginger – Daily Zing shot
5g carbs Orange Ginger Cayenne Shot
4g carbs Wheatgrass Shot
2g carbs Wheatgrass Detox Shot

2g carbs 3G Charger Super Boost

http://www.jambajuice.com/menu-and-nutrition/menu/tasty-bites/breakfast-wraps-sandwiches

4. CHICKEN

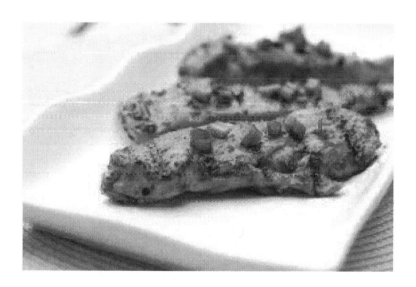

CHICKEN HACKS FROM DIRTY, LAZY, KETO:

*Grilled is better than fried.

*Choose the option with the least amount of breading and pull off any breading that is served on your chicken.

*Stick with the bone-in wings. They are usually not breaded and much lower in carbs than the boneless wings.

*Baked/grilled wings are preferred, but with only a dry rub or thin coating of sauce - not fried.

*Boneless wings are just a marketing gimmick – "chicken nuggets for adults". They are made up of breast meat that is whole meat or ground, breaded, and fried in the shape of a wing. Don't be fooled.

*In general, choose a drier rub for your wings as that has less carbs than a "wet" rub. I'm sure this goes without saying, but I recommend you inspect your wings for any breading that could sneak into your order and may not have been disclosed on the menu. How many times have you gotten an onion ring with your fries by accident? Always be vigilant.

CHICK-FIL-A: HACKS FROM THE AUTHORS OF DIRTY, LAZY, KETO

Stephanie suggests NOT going there on Sundays. They're closed! Upon researching this book, Stephanie was sad to see that all of

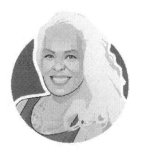

her favorite menu items were completely out of control -- too many carbs! With that realization under her belt, next time Stephanie will order a Chick-fil-A® Chicken Sandwich without the bread. The filet looks to be a good size and the chicken here is always good. She is still sad about her beloved Cobb Salad, though, so this will take some getting over.

Bill loves to eat the Grilled Chicken Nuggets. They are fantastic dipped in ranch dressing. It's like being a kid again in the cafeteria, but much healthier!

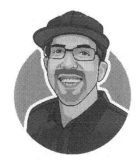

Lastly, we award Chick-fil-A a sad face for not meeting our low carb needs. Their online nutritional information was cumbersome to use, and we hope they will expand their low carb menu.

CHICK-FIL-A: 10 CARBS OR LESS

BREAKFAST
0g carbs Grilled Chick-fil-A Breakfast Filet
2g carbs Grilled Chicken, Egg & Cheese Bagel, no bread
3g carbs Sausage, Egg and Cheese Biscuit, no bread
1g carbs Egg White Grill, no bread
1g carbs side order of Scrambled Eggs

Drinks
0g carbs Large THRIVE Farmer's Coffee

LUNCH
3g carbs Lettuce Wrapped Grilled Chicken Sandwich
3g carbs Grilled Chicken Club Sandwich, no bread
8g carbs Chick-fil-A® Chicken Sandwich, no bread

Strips and Nuggets
1g carbs 4-piece Grilled Chicken Nuggets
2g carbs 6-piece Grilled Chicken Nuggets
2g carbs 8-piece Grilled Chicken Nuggets
3g carbs 12-piece Grilled Chicken Nuggets
4g carbs 4-piece Chicken Nuggets
6g carbs 6-piece Chicken Nuggets
8g carbs 8-piece Chicken Nuggets
7g carbs 1 Piece Chick-n-Strips

10g carbs Fruit Cup (Medium)

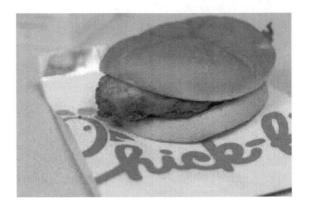

Dips
6g carbs Chick-fil-A Sauce
1g carbs Garlic and Herb Ranch Sauce
10g carbs Siracha Sauce
1g carbs Zesty Buffalo Sauce
10g carbs BBQ Sauce

Salads- no Dressing
6g carbs Grilled Market Salad, no fruit, no granola
7g carbs Spicy Southwest Salad, no corn, no black beans, no pepitas, no tortilla strips
7g carbs Cobb Salad w/ Grilled Chicken, no corn, no honey
3g carbs Side Salad w/o Toppings
9g carbs Side Salad w/ Toppings
7g carbs Chicken Salad Cup

Dressings
2g carbs Creamy Salsa Dressing
3g carbs Light Italian Dressing
3g carbs Light Balsamic Dressing
2g carbs Garlic and Herb Ranch Dressing
3g carbs Avocado Lime Ranch Dressing
1g carbs Chili Lime Vinaigrette Dressing

Drinks

0g carbs Medium Coffee
0g carbs Diet Coke®
0g carbs Large Unsweetened Iced Tea

https://www.chick-fil-a.com/

KFC: HACKS FROM THE AUTHORS OF **DIRTY, LAZY, KETO**

Stephanie suggests mixing hot sauce with ranch dressing as a dip for your chicken. "Finger Linkin' Good!"

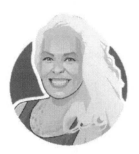

Bill fondly remembers his pre-keto years of eating a bucket of Kentucky FRIED chicken. Oh, those were the days! Now that the restaurant has rebranded themselves to be just KFC, they have thrown a bone to us low carb eaters. Thank you, KFC, for the grilled chicken options!

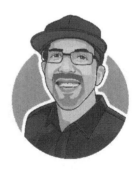

KFC: 10 Carbs or Less

BREAKFAST
No Breakfast Served

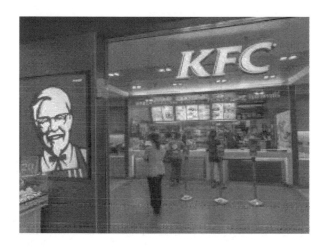

LUNCH
0g carbs Grilled Drumstick
0g carbs Grilled Thigh
0g carbs Grilled Breast
3g carbs Original Recipe Drumstick
7g carbs Original Recipe Thigh
9g carbs Original Recipe Breast
8g carbs Zinger Sandwich, no Bun

2g carbs Side of Green Beans

Dips
2g carbs Buttermilk Ranch Dipping Sauce Cup
0g carbs Colonel's Buttery Spread

2g carbs Creamy Buffalo Dipping Sauce Cup
5g carbs Finger Lickin' Good™ Dipping Sauce Cup
9g carbs Grape Jelly Packet
6g carbs Honey Mustard Dipping Sauce Cup
8g carbs Honey Sauce Packet
8g carbs Ketchup
1g carbs Lemon Juice Packet
9g carbs Strawberry Jam Packet
9g carbs Summertime BBQ Dipping Sauce Cup

Salads
1g carbs Caesar Side Salad, no Dressing
1g carbs House Side Salad, no dressing
1g carbs Heinz Buttermilk Dressing
4g carbs Creamy Parmesan Caesar Dressing

Drinks
0g carbs Diet Pepsi®
0g carbs Diet Dr. Pepper®
1g carbs Diet Mtn. Dew®
0g carbs Diet Mist Twist®
0g carbs Diet Wild Cherry Pepsi®
0g carbs Lipton® Brisk No Calorie Peach Iced Green Tea

https://www.kfc.com/nutrition/full-nutrition-guide

POPEYES: HACKS FROM THE AUTHORS OF DIRTY, LAZY, KETO

Stephanie loves the Blackened Tenders with a side of green beans. Spicy and filling!

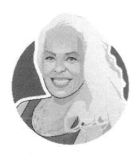

Bill would like to see their low carb menu expanded. Right now, it's slim pickins at Popeyes.

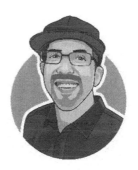

POPEYES: 10 CARBS OR LESS

BREAKFAST

0g carbs Side order of Scrambled Eggs
3g carbs Sausage Biscuit, no bread
3g carbs Egg and Sausage Biscuit, no bread

0g carbs Unsweetened Coffee

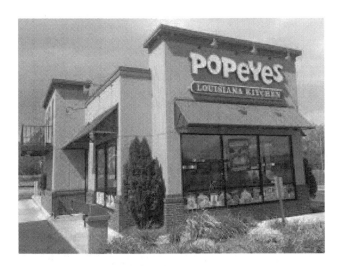

LUNCH/DINNER

2g carbs 3 Piece Blackened Chicken Tenders
3g carbs 5 Piece Blackened Chicken Tenders
4g carbs Bonafide Chicken Drumstick
6g carbs Bonafide Fried Chicken Thigh
6g carbs Blackened Chicken Tender Po'boy Sandwich, no bread

Sides and Sauces
5g carbs Side of Green Beans
2g carbs 1 ounce Blackened Ranch Sauce
3g carbs 1 ounce Buttermilk Ranch

Drinks
0g carbs Diet Pepsi®
0g carbs Diet Coke®
0g carbs Unsweetened Tea

https://popeyes.com/menu/nutrition-information/

Church's: Hacks from the Authors of DIRTY, LAZY, KETO

Stephanie suggests going to a different restaurant. Why should we pay money for food then have to peel off all the breading and hope that unwanted carbs don't slip through? That's just wrong people. Church's, please add some grilled chicken to your menu!

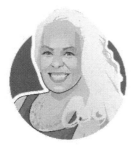

Bill adores jalapeños, so he is going to cut Church's some slack. Who doesn't love the idea

of free whole jalapeños served with your meal? He is willing to get down and dirty with his chicken peeling in order to enjoy this spicy treat.

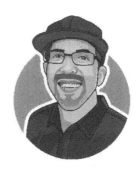

Even though Bill and Stephanie disagree on this one, she is single-handedly awarding the sad face to Church's Chicken. No one should be getting their hands dirty — that's disgusting!

CHURCH'S: 10 CARBS OR LESS

BREAKFAST
3g carbs Sausage Egg and Cheese Biscuit, no bread
1g carbs Steak Biscuit, no bread, no sauce
3g carbs Breakfast Biscuit, no bread
3g carbs Bacon, Egg and Cheese Biscuit, no bread

Drinks
0g carbs 12 oz Coffee, unsweetened

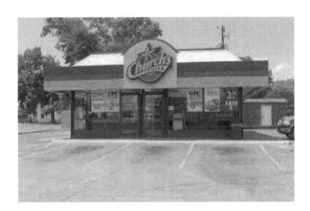

LUNCH
2g carbs Fried Drumsticks (Partially Peeled), Original Recipe
4g carbs Fried Chicken Thighs (Partially Peeled), Original Recipe
3g carbs Fried Chicken Breast (Partially Peeled), Original Recipe
6g carbs Fried Drumsticks, Original Recipe
10g carbs Fried Chicken Thighs, Original Recipe
9g carbs Fried Chicken Breast, Original Recipe
5g carbs Tender Strip (1)
1g carb Jalapeño (1)

6g carbs 1 Boneless Wing, no sauce
2g carbs Cheeseburger, no bread
5g carbs Side of Green Beans

Sauces
4g carbs Honey Mustard Sauce
2g carbs Ranch Sauce
2g carbs Creamy Jalapeño Sauce
2g carbs Ketchup
1g carbs Texas Pete® Hot Sauce
3g carbs Tartar Sauce
6g carbs Cocktail Sauce

Drinks
0g carbs Diet Coke®
0g carbs Large Unsweetened Tea
0g carbs Diet Dr. Pepper®
4g carbs Large Minute Maid Light Lemonade®
0g carbs Large Gold Peak Unsweetened Black Tea

https://www.churchs.com/downloads/nutrition/Nutitional_Information
.pdf

WING STOP: HACKS FROM THE AUTHORS OF DIRTY, LAZY, KETO

Stephanie loves the fact that this restaurant serves celery. CELERY at a fast food restaurant is practically unheard of! Ask your server to bring you a side of celery with your wing order and enjoy the meal dipped with ranch or blue cheese dressing.

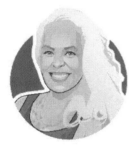

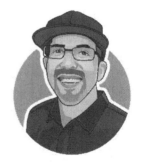

Bill's recommendation: DO NOT order the Boneless Wings or Boneless Tenders, as they are breaded and loaded with carbs. Instead, order the "Jumbo Wings" that are "bone-in" and not breaded. Some of the sauces are high in carbs, so be mindful about your sauce selection.

Wing Stop: 10 Carbs or Less

BREAKFAST
No Breakfast Served

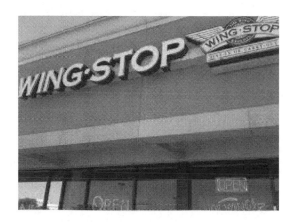

LUNCH/DINNER
1g carbs 2 pc Plain Jumbo Wings
2g carbs 2 pc Atomic Jumbo Wings
1g carbs 2 pc Cajun Jumbo Wings
1g carbs 2 pc Original Hot Jumbo Wings
1g carbs 2 pc Garlic Parmesan Jumbo Wings
1g carbs 2 pc Louisiana Rub Jumbo Wings
1g carbs Veggie Sticks (celery) 4 sticks
3g carbs Veggie Sticks (carrot) 4 sticks

Dressings
2g carbs Ranch 3.25 oz cup
3g carbs Blue Cheese 3.25 oz cup

Drinks

0g carbs Diet Coke®
1g carbs Large Lipton® Iced Tea, unsweetened
2g carbs Gold Peak® Unsweetened Tea

https://www.wingstop.com/wp-content/uploads/2018/09/WSR18-0009-Corporate-NutritionalGuide-JumboWings-HR.pdf

Buffalo Wild Wings: Hacks from the Authors of Dirty, Lazy, Keto

Stephanie likes the variety of salads offered by Buffalo Wild Wings. These are fantastic when paired with an order of wings. When

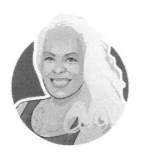

choosing a dressing or sauce for your meal, here is a tip: creamy ranch or blue cheese tend to run lowest in carbs.

Bill's Hacks:
Choose the medium size wings (approx.14) to get a lot of wings for barely any carbs. Of course, you can get a smaller portion for less carbs.

Don't be fooled by the healthy sounding choices that are not healthy AT ALL. For example, the Buffalo Wild Wings has a Southwestern Black Bean Burger that has 22 carbs in the patty alone. HOT DAMN!

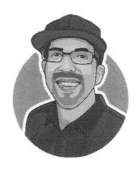

BUFFALO WILD WINGS: 10 CARBS OR LESS

BREAKFAST
No Breakfast Served Most locations

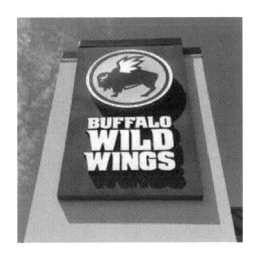

LUNCH/DINNER

Wings

4g carbs Traditional Medium Bone-In Wings (Approx. 14) Blazin' Sauce

4g carbs Traditional Medium Bone-in Wings (Approx. 14) Medium Sauce

5g carbs Traditional Medium Bone-in Wings (Approx. 14) Parmesan Garlic Sauce

5g carbs Traditional Medium Bone-in Wings (Approx. 14) Spicy Garlic Sauce

5g carbs Traditional Medium Bone-in Wings (Approx. 14) Wild Sauce

1g carbs Traditional Medium Bone-in Wings (Approx. 14) Buffalo Sauce
3g carbs Traditional Medium Bone-in Wings (Approx. 14) Desert Heat Sauce

Sauces-Sides
3g carbs Mild Buffalo Sauce
4g carbs Medium Buffalo Sauce
5g carbs Hot Buffalo Sauce
2g carbs Blue Cheese Sauce
2g carbs Ranch Sauce

Burgers and Steak
0g carbs Chicken Breast, Grilled, a la carte
1g carbs Cheeseburger, no bread
7g carbs Boston Lager Burger, no bread
5g carbs Buffalo Blue Burger with Light sauce, no bread
4g carbs Screamin' Nacho Burger, no bread, no chips
6g carbs Grilled Steak and Cheese sandwich, no bread

Chicken Sandwiches
5g carbs Grilled Cali Chicken Sandwich, no bread
2g carbs Classic Grilled Chicken Wrap, no tortilla
5g carbs BBQ Grilled Chicken Sandwich, no bread, no BBQ sauce

Sides
1g carbs Celery Sticks - 5 ea.
3g carbs Celery & Carrot Sticks - 5 ea.
2g carbs Blue Cheese Dressing - 1.5 fl. oz.
2g carbs Ranch Dressing - 1.5 fl. oz

Salads- no Dressing
4g carbs Garden Salad, no croutons, no bread stick, no pickled red onions
7g carbs Grilled Chicken Garden Salad, no croutons, no bread stick
6g carbs Grilled Chicken Santa Fe Salad, no tortillas, no corn, no tortilla strips
2g carbs Side Salad, no bread stick, no croutons
3g carbs Caesar Side Salad, no bread stick, no croutons

Dressings
5g carbs BBQ Ranch Dressing - 2 oz
2g carbs Blue Cheese Dressing - 2 oz
3g carbs Buffalo Blue Cheese Dressing - 2 oz
3g carbs Cilantro Lime Ranch Dressing - 2 oz
3g carbs Lemon Vinaigrette - 2 oz
2g carbs Ranch Dressing - 2 oz
2g carbs Southwestern Ranch Dressing - 2 oz

Drinks
0g carbs Diet Pepsi®
1g carbs Diet Mtn. Dew®
0g carbs Unsweetened Iced Tea®

https://www.buffalowildwings.com/globalassets/pdfs/zone-3-2018---nutrition-guide-1.pdf

5. CHINESE

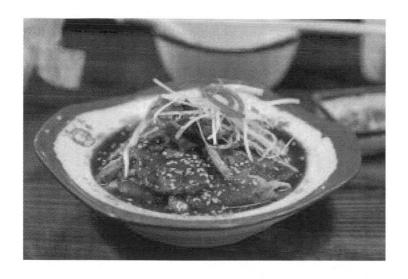

CHINESE FOOD HACKS FROM DIRTY, LAZY, KETO:

*Beware of the sauces. There are lots of carbs in the sweet sauces due to added sugar.

*Avoid rice or noodles. Choose steamed veggies as your side.

*Soy sauce, depending on brand, may contain carbs (0-3 carbs per Tbsp.), so be sure to include this in your meal planning.

*Go spicy instead of sweet - adding wasabi adds strong flavor without adding carbs.

PANDA EXPRESS: HACKS FROM THE AUTHORS OF DIRTY, LAZY, KETO

Stephanie suggests ordering the Grilled Teriyaki Chicken, though it's hefty in carbs. The mixed veggie option goes well with the chicken.

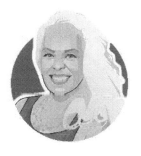

Be wary of portion size at Panda Express. The nutritional information is for the serving size listed, but we have noticed the staff ladles inconsistent amounts onto plates and to-go containers. You might accidently eat way too many

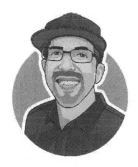

carbs due to this variability.

Bill's recommendation is to pass on this restaurant. For the amount of carbs in such a small serving, you are likely to walk away still hungry.

PANDA EXPRESS: 10 CARBS OR LESS

BREAKFAST
No Breakfast Served

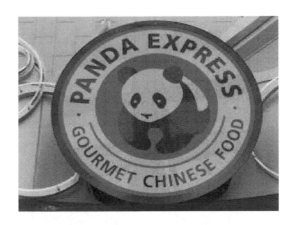

LUNCH/DINNER
8g carbs Grilled Teriyaki Chicken, 6 oz. serving
8g carbs Grilled Asian Chicken, 6 oz serving
9g carbs String Bean Chicken Breast, 6 oz. serving
10g carbs Mushroom Chicken, 6 oz. serving
8g carbs Hot Szechuan Tofu, 5.5 oz. serving
8g carbs Steamed Ginger Fish, 6 oz. serving
10g carbs Kung Pao Chicken, 4.4 oz. serving
5g carbs Mixed Veggies, Entree
8g carbs Country Style Bean Curd, 4 oz. serving

Sauces
2g carbs Chili Sauce 1 Packet (7g)
0g carbs Soy Sauce 1 Packet (6g)

3g carbs Pot Sticker Sauce 1 Packet
0g carbs Hot Mustard 1 Packet (7g)
3g carbs Plum Sauce 1 Packet (7g)

Drinks
0g carbs Diet Pepsi®
0g carbs Lipton® No Calorie Brisk Peach Iced Tea
0g carbs China Mist Iced Tea®

https://www.pandaexpress.com/

ONO HAWAIIAN BBQ: HACKS FROM THE AUTHORS OF DIRTY, LAZY, KETO

Stephanie likes pretending she is in Hawaii while sitting in the strip mall at Ono Hawaiian BBQ. The cute décor is distracting, and it's fun to have some different flavors for lunch.

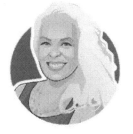

Bill likes the variety of lunch items here, as long as he is strong willed enough to pass on the carbolicious macaroni salad that seems to

come with every meal. The cashiers are great about heaping on extra servings of cabbage instead of the steamed rice, so that helps to bulk up his meal on the cheap.

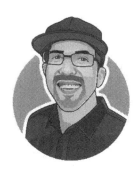

Despite offering cabbage, we are awarding a sad face to ONO HAWAIIAN BBQ as they are not meeting our low carb needs. They don't even have the nutritional information chart on their website! We had to email them directly to get a copy. Come on guys, help us out!

ONO HAWAIIAN BBQ: 10 CARBS OR LESS

BREAKFAST
No Breakfast Served

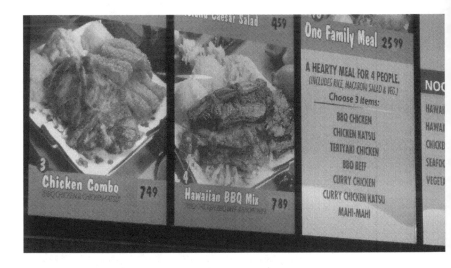

LUNCH/DINNER
Aloha Plate Pick One Choice (Sides not included)
5g carbs Lemon Pepper Chicken
0g carbs Grilled Chicken Breast
9g carbs Teriyaki Chicken
9g carbs Hawaiian BBQ Chicken
8g carbs Beef Short Rib, no sauce
4g carbs Kalua Pork with Cabbage

Mini Meals (Sides not included)
7g carbs Island Curry Chicken Mini Meal

3g carbs Lemon Pepper Chicken Mini Meal
7g carbs Hawaiian BBQ Chicken Mini Meal
6g carbs Teriyaki Chicken Mini Meal, No Sauce
0g carbs Grilled Chicken Breast

Aloha Plate Pick Two Choices (Sides not included)
2g carbs Grilled Chicken Breast + Kalua Pork
6g carbs Grilled Chicken Breast + BBQ Beef
9g carbs BBQ Chicken + Teriyaki Chicken
9g carbs BBQ Chicken + Island Curry Chicken
5g carbs BBQ Chicken + Grilled Chicken Breast
7g carbs BBQ Chicken + Kalua Pork
9g carbs Teriyaki Chicken + Island Curry Chicken
5g carbs Teriyaki Chicken + Grilled Chicken Breast
5g carbs Island Curry Chicken + Grilled Chicken Breast

Sides
6g carbs Serving of Cabbage, 4 oz

Salads
6g carbs Fresh Mix Side Salad, 4 oz

Drinks
Vary by location

http://www.onohawaiianbbq.com/menu/ono-plate-lunches/

6. PIZZA

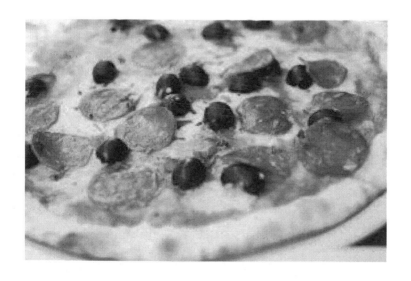

PIZZA HACKS From DIRTY, LAZY, KETO:

*Go crustless! Pull the toppings off a slice of pizza and throw away the crust.

*Most pizza restaurants serve chicken wings (baked/grilled, not deep-fried) or side salads. Both of these options are keto friendly!

*Avoid the BBQ wings and the pineapple topping. Both are sweet and full of carbs.

*We've read hacks on the internet about trying to order a pizza without the crust, asking the employees to use a strong foundation of cheese as the base instead. First of all, that sounds like a lot of work for the employees and a potential fire hazard. Second, do you really want to eat that much cheese?

*Recently, we have seen a few pizza chains offer a cauliflower crust option. This is exciting news! Just this week I saw advertisements from Pizza Rev and California Pizza Kitchen with this reference. The carb counts were still too high for our preferences, but I would like to acknowledge that they are TRYING! There is hope for all of us pizza fans.

*Pizza is a tough category for those of us that follow a DIRTY, LAZY, KETO diet. In fact, Italian food, in general, is known for being just too carbolicious! If pizza, pasta, and breadsticks are a weakness of yours, it might be easier to steer clear of the pizza restaurants altogether. Know thyself!

*Lastly, we wouldn't be able to sleep tonight if we didn't offer the "Fat Head Pizza Crust" recipe here. This popular pizza dough alternative might help with your pizza cravings! Share this recipe with your local pizzerias with the hope of influencing their menu.

FAT HEAD PIZZA CRUST

Share with your local pizzeria with hopes they add a low-carb crust to their menu!

INGREDIENTS:

1 ½ cups shredded mozzarella cheese
¾ cup almond flour (9 net carbs if using Bob's Red Mill)
2 tbsp cream cheese
1 egg beaten
garlic powder to taste

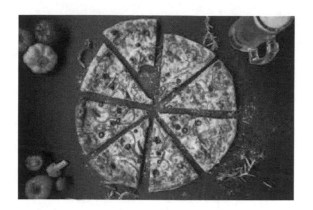

Instructions:

1. Put mozzarella and cream cheese in a microwaveable bowl and heat for one minute. Stir and replace in microwave for another 30 seconds.
2. Stir in beaten egg and flour.
3. Wet hands and spread dough thin on parchment paper. Spread evenly. (If the dough is stringy, then the cheese has hardened too much. Microwave again to soften.)
4. Poke rows of holes with a fork to avoid bubbling when cooking the dough.
5. Sprinkle the dough with garlic powder.
6. Bake 425F (pre heated) for about 10-12 minutes or until slightly brown on top. (Poke holes in any bubbles that form while this is cooking.) Your dough is ready!
7. Top with your favorite toppings and return to bake in oven for 8-10 minutes until your cheese browns. Enjoy!

LITTLE CAESARS: HACKS FROM THE AUTHORS OF DIRTY, LAZY, KETO

Stephanie suggests ordering the oven roasted wings and/or salad. Eating only a meal full of melted cheese pulled off the tops of pizza slices isn't satisfying. Plus, it's gross.

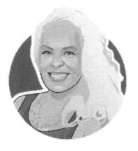

Bill is a huge fan of Little Caesars. The $5 Hot and Ready is a staple in the Laska household. The kids are able to

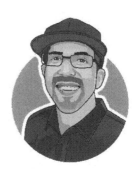

get their pizza fix while the parents sample the Buffalo Caesar Wings. Who doesn't love a drive thru pizza? And the price is just too good to pass up!

LITTLE CAESARS: 10 CARBS OR LESS

BREAKFAST
No breakfast Served

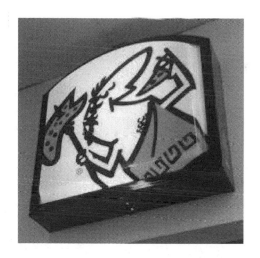

LUNCH/DINNER
2g carbs Hot-N-Ready Pepperoni Classic Round Pizza, Crustless
6g carbs Hot-N-Ready Ultimate Supreme Classic Round Pizza, Crustless

Toppings (Deep! Deep! Dish Size Pizza)
2g carbs Peperoni
0g carbs Bacon
1g carbs Beef
1g carbs Sausage
3g carbs Ham
3g carbs Canadian Bacon

3g carbs Green Pepper
8g carbs Onion
3g carbs Mushroom, Canned
3g carbs Mushroom, Fresh
0g carbs Black Olive
0g carbs Jalapeño Peppers
1g carbs Mild Banana Pepper
4g carbs Extra Cheese

Wings
3g carbs 8 pc Oven Roasted Caesar Wings
3g carbs 8 pc Buffalo Caesar Wings
7g carbs 8 pc Garlic Parmesan Caesar Wings

Sauces (1 Container)
5g carbs Crazy Sauce
3g carbs Cheesy Jalapeño
4g carbs Ranch
3g carbs Buffalo Ranch
0g carbs Butter Garlic Flavor

Salad
6g carbs Antipasto Salad
8g carbs Greek Salad

https://littlecaesars.com/en-us/our-menu/nutrition/

DOMINO'S PIZZA: HACKS FROM THE AUTHORS OF DIRTY, LAZY, KETO

Stephanie suggests enjoying a salad, wings and even the "toppings" of a pizza slice to feel like you are getting the full Domino's experience.

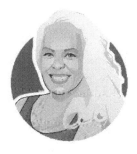

Bill's recommendation: Order the Baked Plain Wings with Kicker Hot Sauce along with the Classic Garden Salad and

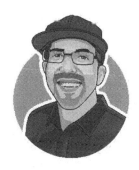

Marzetti Garden Ranch Dressing (no croutons). That ought to fill you up.

Lastly, we would like to award Domino's Pizza with a DIRTY, LAZY, KETO GOLD STAR for their easy to use nutritional guide! We were impressed that their nutritional information even provided carb counts for the crust alone, making it easy to calculate eating "just the toppings." Thanks!

DOMINO'S: 10 CARBS OR LESS

BREAKFAST
No Breakfast Served

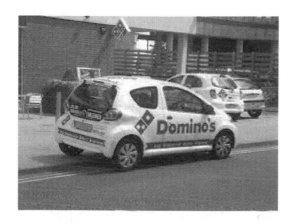

LUNCH/DINNER
Toppings (16 in Extra Large Pizza)
1g carbs American Cheese
2g carbs Bacon
0g carbs Beef
1g carbs Black Olives
0g carbs Cheddar
1g carbs Chicken Grilled
1g carbs Green Peppers
1g carbs Ham
0g carbs Jalapeño
1g carbs Mushrooms
1g carbs Onions
1g carbs Pepperoni
0g carbs Salami
0g carbs Sausage

0g carbs Shredded Parmesan
0g carbs Spinach
1g carbs Diced Tomatoes
0g carbs Hot Sauce

Sauce (16 in Extra Large Pizza)
2g carbs Pizza Sauce
1g carbs Alfredo Sauce
6g carbs BBQ
1g carbs Garlic Parmesan (White Sauce)

Cheese Options (16 in Extra Large Pizza)
3g carbs Regular Cheese
2g carbs Light Cheese
3g carbs Extra Cheese
4g carbs Double Cheese

Wings
7g carbs 4-count of Baked Plain Wings
7g carbs 4-count of Fire Wings
7g carbs 4-count of Hot Wings
8g carbs 4-count of Mild Wings

Sandwiches
6g carbs Italian Baked Sandwich, no bread, no banana peppers or green peppers.
6g carbs Philly Cheese Steak, no bread, no green peppers
4g carbs Italian Sandwich, no bread
3g carbs Mediterranean Veggie Sandwich, no bread

Salads with No Dressing
6g carbs Classic Garden Salad, no croutons
6g carbs Chicken Caesar Salad, no croutons

Dressings
1g carbs Marzetti Cardini Caesar Dressing
2g carbs Marzetti Garden Ranch Dressing
2g carbs Ken's Caesar Dressing

https://www.dominos.com/en/pages/content/nutritional/nutrition.jsp?lang=en

Pizza Hut: Hacks from the Authors of **DIRTY, LAZY, KETO**

Stephanie likes to order the Garlic Parmesan Wings if she is forced to eat at Pizza Hut. The smell of the pizza here is amazing and hard to resist. She prefers to drive away FAST with her "take out" wings in order to avoid a keto dine-in disaster of losing all self-control and ordering bread sticks.

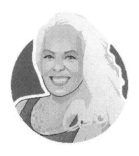

Bill says there are no surprises here. At Pizza Hut, your options are limited. Basically, you can

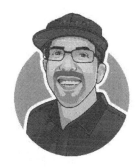

scrape off the cheese and toppings to eat as your meal or order an entrée of wings. They don't even have salads on their menu. How sad!

Lastly, we award a sad face to Pizza Hut for their lack of menu choices and poor online nutritional information.

PIZZA HUT: 10 CARBS OR LESS

BREAKFAST
No Breakfast in Most Locations

3g carbs Bacon, Egg and Cheese Biscuit, no bread
3g carbs Egg and Cheese Biscuit, no bread
2g carbs Sausage Biscuit, no bread

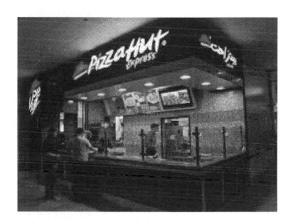

LUNCH/DINNER
Wings
0g carbs 6 Bone in All American Wings, not crispy
3g carbs 6 Bone-In Garlic Parmesan Wings, not crispy
8g carbs 2 Buffalo Mild Wings, not crispy
8g carbs 2 Buffalo Medium Wings, not crispy
8g carbs 2 Buffalo Burnin' Hot Wings, not crispy

Pizza
6g carbs Medium Supreme Pizza, no crust. May have to scrape the toppings off the crust.

7g carbs Large Meat Lover's Pizza, crustless

Sauce
2g carbs Ranch Dipping Sauce, 1.5 oz

https://m.nutritionix.com/pizza-hut/menu/premium/

7. SEAFOOD

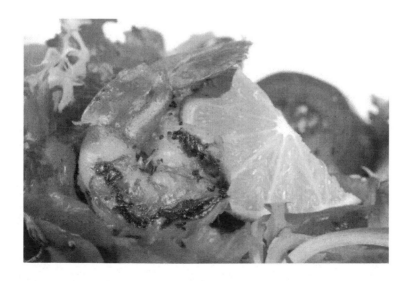

SEAFOOD HACKS FROM DIRTY, LAZY, KETO

*Baked items are better! Anything breaded will be higher in carbs.

*Be careful with the sweet sauces like "Sweet Thai Chili Sauce" and "Sweet and Sour Sauce" as those are full of added sugar.

*Go spicy instead of sweet. Adding hot sauce to your seafood will bring more flavor.

LONG JOHN SILVER'S: HACKS FROM THE AUTHORS OF DIRTY, LAZY, KETO

Stephanie orders one piece of Baked Cod with malt vinegar, broccoli and green beans. It's a hearty, hot meal for 8 carbs!

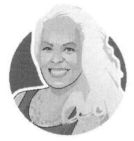

Bill is a fan of the battered shrimp. What a fun splurge to enjoy fried food on keto!

It's cool that Long John Silver's has hung on for so long. This "old school" restaurant brings me back to my childhood. It's fun to have seafood as a fast-food option for variety.

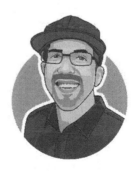

LONG JOHN SILVER'S: 10 CARBS OR LESS

BREAKFAST
No Breakfast Served

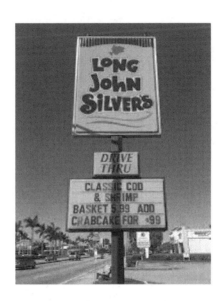

LUNCH/DINNER
7g carbs 1 Crispy Breaded Chicken Tender
0g carbs 3 pc. Baked Shrimp
5g carbs 3 pc. Battered Shrimp
1g carbs Baked Cod, 1 piece
8g carbs Battered Cod, 1 piece
3g carbs Baked Cod with Garlic Butter (2 pieces)
0g carbs Baked Salmon, 1 piece

Sides
4g carbs Broccoli (individual size)
9g carbs 3 Piece Broccoli Cheese Bites
3g carbs Seasoned Green Beans (Individual Size)

Sauces
4g carbs Cocktail Sauce 1 dipping cup
1g carbs Creamy Garlic Butter Sauce 1 oz.
1g carbs Creamy Ranch Dressing 1 packet
2g carbs Honey Mustard Sauce 1 packet
8g carbs Ketchup 1 pouch
0g carbs Lemon Juice 1 packet
0g carbs Louisiana Hot Sauce 1 teaspoon
0g carbs Malt Vinegar 0.5 oz.
4g carbs Marinara
3g carbs Tartar Sauce 1 packet

Drinks
2g carbs 12oz coffee, unsweetened
0g carbs Diet Pepsi®
0g carbs Diet Dr. Pepper®
0g carbs Silver's® Iced Tea (unsweetened)
0g carbs Brick Peach® Iced Green Tea

https://docs.wixstatic.com/ugd/1fbc3f_161fa148e1f24f8fb00208871d70d0d8.pdf

8. FINAL WORDS

••

We hope you enjoyed your journey with <u>DIRTY, LAZY, KETO Fast Food Guide: Ten Carbs or Less.</u>

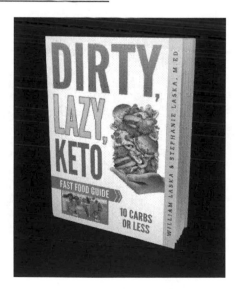

We would be so thankful if you gave us an honest review in Amazon! It's so easy to do. You don't even need to write anything fancy, just click the stars. You can even post a review anonymously. Your neighbors will never know how much you enjoy fast food!

Your review helps other readers find the book on Amazon. Books will lots of reviews tend to "float to the top". This helps other readers find the book and ultimately helps our chosen charity, Goodwill.

Not sure how to do this? Simply log into your Amazon account, find the book title, click on the stars and then "leave a review." Simple, and so helpful!

Lastly, your reviews and feedback are so motivating to Stephanie and Bill! We are passionate about helping you improve your eating, and want to keep writing books about this topic. Those little gold stars matter A LOT to our family. In fact, we read your Amazon reviews aloud around the dinner table.

While you are shopping on Amazon, don't forget to order your copy of <u>DIRTY, LAZY, KETO Getting Started: How I Lost 140 Pounds</u> by Stephanie Laska.

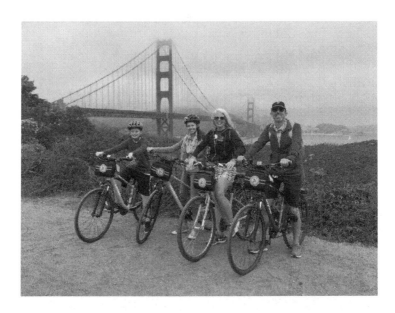

If you would like to receive FREE ongoing articles and tips to help you in your weight loss journey, register your email at http://DirtyLazyKeto.com

Join other fans of the DIRTY, LAZY, KETO community by joining the free author-led Facebook group:

http://facebook.com/groups/dirtylazyketo

For continued social media updates about DIRTY, LAZY, KETO follow us at:

https://twitter.com/140lost
https://www.instagram.com/140lost/
https://www.facebook.com/DIRTYLAZYKETO

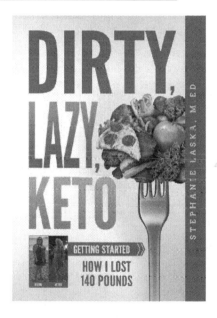

Made in the USA
San Bernardino, CA
27 March 2019